Tiredness, Chronic Fatigue & Exhaustion

Neurophysiology and Cardiovascular Risk

Dr David H. Dighton

MediCause

Published by MediCause.

British Library Cataloguing in Publication Data

A CIP catalogue record for this title is available from the British Library

Hardback ISBN: 978-1-0683597-3-6

e-book ISBN: 978-1-0683597-7-4

115 High Rd., Loughton. Essex. IG10 4JA UK.

+44(0)2085087741 david@daviddighton.com

Dedication

For all those who spent their energy encouraging me.

I am indebted to one cardiologist, Dr. Peter Nixon, who provided me with insight into the psycho-social origins of cardiac ill-health, and how its reversal can reduce risk.

Few possess insightful providence; insight which brings the light of understanding to knowledge, extinguishing the darkness of ignorance.
New ideas can disturb those with fixed ideas, those with vested interests, and those whose claim to fame is based on half-truth or spurious validity. They will work hard to reject the acceptance of contrary ideas. This book is based on what I learned about human nature from a man of insight. With Peter Nixon as my teacher at Charing Cross Hospital, London, in the 1970s, I learned not only about the plight of men pregnant with new ideas, but how the establishment can treat them, should they remain non-conformist.

From Peter Nixon, I learned how ill-health, and in particular cardiac ill-health, can arise from the fatigue caused by discordant relationships and the life circumstances that influence them. I learned how highly motivated humans can get injured and suffer illness; how their energy can be harnessed to restore their health through experience-based advice, evidence-based medical care, and constructive counselling, and how we might reduce the risk of some medical catastrophes.

About the Author

Formerly,

British Heart Foundation Research Fellow,
St. George's Hospital, London.
Lecturer in Cardiology,
Charing Cross Hospital, London.
Chef de Clinique, Cardiologist. Vrije Universiteit, Amsterdam.

Director: Cardiac Centre, Loughton, Essex, UK.
Chigwell Cardiac Centre, Essex. UK.
www.daviddighton.com
email:
david@daviddighton.com

Dr. David H. Dighton qualified at the London Hospital Medical College in 1966 with MB and BS (London) degrees. In 1970, after some time spent in an NHS general practice, he became a British Heart Foundation Fellow in Cardiology at St. George's Hospital, Hyde Park Corner, London, working with cardiologists Dr. Aubrey Leatham and Dr. Alan Harris. In 1973, he became a

MRCP(UK), and later a Lecturer (London University) in Medicine and Cardiology at Charing Cross Hospital, London.

In 1980, he became Chef de Clinique (Assistant Professor) at the Vrije University Hospital, Amsterdam. After returning to the UK in 1982, he worked both in his own private medical and cardiac practice in Loughton, Essex (The Loughton Clinic, established in 1973), and at the Wellington Hospital, London. In 2000, he started a private cardiac diagnostic centre, specialising in heart disease prevention and the early detection of heart and artery disease (The Cardiac Centre, Loughton). This closed after the PSA directed the GMC to withdrawn his licence to practice (see the details in 'The NHS. Our Sick Sacred Cow.' 2023). As an independent private cardiologist and general physician, he disagreed with them about UK medical practice bureaucracy, and those most qualified to devise, regulate and supervise it; opinions he based on having been a medical student, general physician and cardiologist for sixty years.

In 2003 and 2006, he wrote two books on food and the heart, and between 2023 and 2024, six books on medical and cardiac subjects. He is continuing to publish books on both medical topics and his research relating to secondary cardiac prevention.

One result of his interest in the frontier between art and science, is one small book of poems, haiku and senryu, on inter-personal relationships. His magnum opus, The Art and Science of Medical Practice, details what he learned from practising the art and science of medicine for sixty years.

This is his tenth book, but he has other interests. He draws (all the illustrations in this book) and paints in oils on canvas. He has played the guitar and piano for many decades, for his own amusement. He has composed several simple melodies, one of which introduces his YouTube series on understanding heart problems (Dr. Dighton interviews), another of which he played live (on Facebook) for his now much missed patient and friend, June Robins.

For further information go to: www.daviddighton.com

Email: david@daviddighton.com

Other Works by the Author

Eat to Your Heart's Content. The diet and lifestyle for a healthy heart.(2003). HeartShield.
ISBN: 0-9551072-0-2

HeartSense. How to look after your heart.(2006) . HeartShield.
ISBN: 0-9551072-1-0

The NHS: Our Sick Sacred Cow: Causes and Cures (2023)
Paperback. ISBN: 978-1-3999-6027-4 (also ebook from: https ://stan.store/drdhd001001)

How to Become Heart-Smart. A User's Guide to Hear Health and Heart Disease Prevention. (2023 1st Ed./2nd Ed. 2024. ISBN: 978-1-3999-7461-5 (also ebook from: https://stan. store/drdhd001001)

Who Loses Wins. Winning Weight Loss Battles: A 'Fat Mentality' v A 'Fit Mentality' (2024).
Paperback ISBN: 978-1-7385207-1-8; ebook: 978-1-7385207-2-5. (from: https://stan.store/drdhd001001)

Doctors, Nurses & Patients. How to Survive Medical Practice (2024). ISBN: Paperback: 978-1-7385207-5-6; ebook: 978-1-7385207-6-3 ((from: https://stan.store/drdhd001001)

The Art and Science of Medical Practice (2024). ISBN: (hardback: 978-1-7385207-7-0;

Paperback: 978-1-7385207-3-2; ebook: 978-1-7385207-4-9 (from: https://stan.store/drdhd001001)

Poems for Recycling Lives (2024).

ISBN: Paperback: 978-1-7385207-8-7; ebook: 978-1-7385207-9-4

Essential Adult Cardiology. A Textbook for Aspiring Cardiologists.

ISBN: Hardback 978-0683597-0-5; Paperback 978-0683597-2-9; e-book 978-0683597-1-2

Goto: www.daviddighton.com for more information

Contents

Detailed Contents

Chapter 2: Neurobiological Energetics and TFE.

Assumptions and postulates. Arising questions. Cerebral electrical and molecular activity. Data from neuro-imaging. Brain power and EEG waveforms. Mental effort and the EEG. Brain power. Energy considerations and neuronal electrical activity. ATP production and usage.

Chapter 3: Neurotransmitters and TFE symptoms.

Acetylcholine (ACh). Two models of ACh activity. ACh synthesis. Nor-epinephrine (NE). Serotonin. Dopamine. GABA. Glutamate. Melatonin.

Chapter 4: Bio-Physical Neurophysiology.

Electronic circuits comparisons. Switches and synapses. Energy, power, stress, and strain. LCR circuits. Constitution; power, time. Brain circuitry, resistance, capacitance, gates, and pathways. Amplification and suppression. Entropy and catastrophe.

PART TWO: CLINICAL ASPECTS

Chapter 5: Ancient and Modern Views of Sleep: The Divine Panacea?

Depiction and understanding of sleep and dreaming throughout history. Ancient Greek, pre-Socratic, and Hippocratic writers. The Hippocratic text. Coan Prenotions. Psukhē 'On Regimen IV'. Asclepius. Lucretius. Shakespeare. Sculpture and painting. Freud and Jung.

Chapter 6: The Role of Sleep and Sleep Disturbance in TFE.

Effective and ineffective sleep. Phases of 'normal' sleep. Disturbances of normal sleep. Sleep apnoea. REM sleep disorder. Narcolepsy. Somnambulism. Depression. Aging. Traumatic brain injury. The causes of sleep disturbance.. Sleep disorder epidemiology. Clinical significance of disturbed sleep. Claude Bernard: OPHERIC approach. Sleep management. Biological clock. Alcohol, food, and sleep. Sleep surrogates. The Sabbath and biological function. Delegation and resignation of duty. Sleep induction. Sleep hygiene. Drugged sleep. Addiction and withdrawal. The siesta.

Chapter 10: The Clinical Management of TFE.

TFE symptom management. Non-sleep, neurophysiological re-setting. Sleep management. Sleep therapy. Tactical napping. Cognitive behavioural therapy. Hypnosis. Distraction and relaxation. Relevant clinical diagnoses.

PART THREE

Conclusions

'Connectomics'. Fast and slow thinking. Cerebral energy from different scales. Plasticity and synaptic strength. Global cerebral functioning. The perception of energy expenditure. Spartan TFE management.

PostScript

Medical practice management and TFE identification.

Introduction

"It is what we think we already know that often prevents us from learning"

Claude Bernard. 1865.

The personal, social, and economic consequences of chronic tiredness, fatigue, and exhaustion symptoms (TFE) affect many millions of people worldwide, so a better understanding of the origins and treatment is apposite. Since symptoms can vary from mild tiredness to severe exhaustion, and be acute or chronic, I have used the collective term TFE. As a cardiologist, my particular focus has been to relate TFE symptoms to the occurrence of cardiac infarction and stroke, and the management of ischaemic heart disease and hypertension.

TFE symptoms are most commonly referred to as chronic fatigue syndrome or (CFS) or myalgic encephalitis (ME). These nebulous conditions have no single medical cause, but have many negative implications for health, disease, life at home, work efficiency, and sporting prowess. This review examines the psychosocial characteristics, relationship to sleep, possible infective origins, and biochemical and neurophysiological aspects. I suggest its most likely origins and review various treatment options.

Symptoms of TFE are common to the natural history of many diseases, but not always caused by disease. Regardless of the cause, the more extreme the TFE (fatigue and exhaustion), the greater the risk of ill-health, death, accidental injury, or the progression of disease towards a poorer prognosis. To reverse CFS, a complicated strategy may be necessary. This differs from simple tiredness caused by everyday activity, and reversed by one night of refreshing sleep.

In the US, 'fatigue is estimated to cost employers about $136 billion a year in health-related lost productivity' (NSC. US. 2025). Absenteeism, ill-health and more frequent injuries and accidents are sometimes the result. The medical profession often gets involved, and for many reasons, will often prove impotent to help.

Many academic questions about the aetiology of TFE symptoms remain, but answers need to be found if effective solutions are to be made available.

Is tiredness a psychological phenomenon, related only to mood? Are there neurochemical causes at the intracellular molecular level, or alterations in brain neurotransmitters? If neurotransmitters are involved, what has caused them to change? Have some people inherited a neurobiological predisposition to TFE, or are external stresses and insomnia the only causes? This treatise addresses these questions and explores the cardiovascular and other medical consequences of CFS.

Patients suffering with TFE symptoms can dismay members of the medical profession. This is partly because doctors have long known that routine, science-based investigation is often fruitless. Finding a discrete clinical diagnostic cause is uncommon (1.5% in my unpublished series of 1000 cases), so few doctors undertake further engagement. This can leave the patient perplexed and demoralised.

The medical profession in the UK has major problems: over specialisation, anonymity, an ever-increasing lack of personal doctor-patient engagement, and minimal continuity. This means that doctors who never ask patients about their work and family living circumstances, as part of the 'investigations', remain acceptable professionals. Only the few are interested enough to ask: what factors drained the patient's energy?; what reasons underlie patients' inability to replete it, and can we help? Doctors wishing to remain anonymous and following ill-educated managerial dictates that control the time available for each patient, exacerbate the problem of dismissing TFE symptoms.

There is an art to harnessing our personal energy resources, with few masters. Some people seem to 'get it right', although I know from the many confidences vested in me that appearances are often mistaken. To be a long-living fly on the walls of others might help us see the truth. If someone, sometime, does 'get it right', their art and science of life should have discernible features worthy of discovery and understanding. This knowledge could make life mastery accessible.

"If you have talent and energy, you're king. If you have only energy and no talent, you're still a prince. But if you have talent and no energy, you're a pauper."

Jeffrey Archer. 2009.

The personal energy we have, and take for granted until lost, is our most fundamental resource. To master life as a fully functioning human being, one must know how to manage personal energy. Any recognised master of living, whether by nature or education, will have to have mastered energy management.

In the extreme, TFE can be fatal, especially when associated with frailty, or cardiovascular system (CVS) disease. The abandoning of the exhausted and frail still occurs. In his classic work, The Ascent of Man (1975), Jacob Bronowski details how some Bakhtiari tribesmen in Iran, unable to cross the Bazuft River during its spring flood, faced abandonment and death. In other cultures, the family will care for the tired and elderly until they die. In many western cultures, the tired and elderly are more often displaced from their families to live in care homes.

The aim of this book is to examine the origins and fate of everyday personal energy; how we humans get it, save it, spend it, and suffer the lack of it. Without energy, vigour, or vitality, we lose the power to cope and achieve. Without it, some cannot adapt to new environments, and will not fulfil their desired goals. For some, illness will cause fatalities.

If have approached the subject of molecular neurophysiology with the understanding of a cardiologist and amateur electronics hobbyist. I studied elementary electronics at night school in order to build myself a vectorcardiogram. The cost of the components defeated me, so I later borrowed one. Molecular neurophysiology has progressed since I first became interested in TFE during the 1970s. I have summarised the research findings, pertinent to TFE symptoms, in several early chapters.

Some academic articles state that the purpose of sleep remains obscure, apart from basic restorative physiological functions (Freiberg, A.S. 2020). From a clinical point of view, it has an undoubted role in patient recovery, whether from diseases like cardiac infarction or pneumonia, or the healing of physical damage like hip fracture. Failure to sleep can impede recovery in those who cannot sleep well, although prolonged sleep and lack of activity itself can bring complications like deep vein thrombosis and pneumonia. Unfortunately, data confirming the relationship of sleep to recovery is scarce (Karndar, B.B. et al. 2012).

Some animals like urchins, sponges and jellyfish have no brain, no central nervous system, and do not sleep. Some animals like dolphins and orca, maintain antipredation vigilance with unihemispheric sleep (Mascetti.G.G. 2016). Bullfrogs are thought not to sleep but have dormant periods. Bluefish are also thought not to sleep, but no studies of their neurophysiology and brain chemistry has been undertaken to help us understand sleep and TFE symptoms.

In this treatise, I describe the way humans use energy to bring health and success in life. Disease induction and disease escalation are other aspects of energy management to be considered. The unifying principles of the processes involved must comply with established physical laws, whether applied to humans or the entire universe.

A stress to one person may not be a stress to another, so the concept of stress lacks universal application. This is not so for energy. There can be no understanding of any functioning body without an understanding of its energy requirements and exchanges. The same energy considerations apply to the work needed to maintain our relationships, the cooking of food, chemical reactions, or any human endeavour. Energy is indivisible and universal. We worry about the price of oil, electricity, and gas as energy sources, but give little thought to our personal energy use: its generation, storage, and use for life functioning, be it at a cerebral molecular, or neurophysiological level, or at a metabolic, behavioural or social level.

Both health and success in the business of life (or indeed the life of a business) require effective energy management. Finding energy, keeping it, and knowing how to spend it in order to safeguard health are the subjects of this book. Sleep, relaxation, contentment and joy, seem to sustain our energy, but must be balanced with our spending of energy. Health and disease discussions rarely mention these factors. Instead, the public thinks more of their diet, vitamins, and exercise as the only ingredients for health. Life proceeds, dependent on the maintenance of this balance, since the amount of energy we spend can only ever equal the amount we produce. One problem is that both energy spending and saving energy can be insensible.

In its most fundamental form, all of life and nature depends on a balancing act: between energy expenditure, its production and saving. Because our lives depend on maintaining this energy balance, understanding this life equation is essential to health.

Dickens' Mr Micawber said of money: *'Annual income twenty pounds, annual expenditure nineteen pounds nineteen and six, result happiness. Annual income twenty pounds, annual expenditure twenty pounds nought and six, result misery.'*

Charles Dickens. David Copperfield. 1850.

The same applies to personal energy.

Modern medicine lacks a unifying thesis that relates personal behaviour, attitudes, outlook, the stress we suffer because of our circumstances, environmental challenges, and vital genetic processes, to our energy, health, ill-health, disease, and death. We need a comprehensive thesis to clinically guide energy requirements for coping with and adapting to life, which for some, affects well-known pathological processes including pathogens, immunity, atherosclerosis, blood pressure control, cancer, and mental health.

Considerations of personal energy spending and saving are potent medical factors; factors potent enough to predict our state of health and the onset and progress of pathophysiology.

Many people will suffer unexpected disease throughout their life. Although many result from genetic influence (hypertension, coronary artery disease (CAD), and some cancers), or environmental factors (air pollution, bacteria, and viruses), many suffer ill-health unrelated to disease. They are often victims of a depleted energy status, expressed as tiredness, fatigue, or exhaustion (TFE). We can lose energy by struggling to earn money; in pursuing an acceptable lifestyle and in maintaining meaningful relationships. If poor sleep continues, this energy will not be efficiently repleted. To understand ill-health and its continuance, we must involve energy considerations, just like we must for understanding every action and reaction in the known universe.

Medical professionals rarely consider patient energy status. TFE symptoms can bring dismay to doctors. So much so, they will avoid asking pertinent energy related questions, apart from the calories gained from eating and the energy consumed by exercise. Mental activity is a potent cause of energy loss and TFE. Because it is practically impossible to measure, few physicians consider it. The considerations explored in this treatise should enable a different perspective to the current dismissive outlook.

I learned through having repeated exposure to thousands of patients over many decades that energy considerations are of paramount importance to quality of life, to the control of medical conditions, and to mortality. As perceived energy runs out, and immunity fails, we are more easily overtaken by infection, cardiovascular shock or metastasising cancer. Sometimes the draining of energy results from what Dr. Peter Nixon called 'people poisoning'. It can also result from continuous righteous indignation, resentment, inescapable servitude, indignity, and loss of control. Any mention of these potent clinical factors is usually absent from textbooks of medicine and cardiology.

We can all suffer from an imbalance of personal energy. If we spend more than we save, our capacity for work and rest becomes diminished. In what we perceive as a depleted energy state, we are all liable to biological dysfunction; a state that can lead to reduced resistance to infection, hypertension, mental illness and even hypercoagulability, for those predisposed. Some become exhausted and unable to cope, while others suffer physically. For those who already have coronary atherosclerosis, worsening angina or cardiac infarction can occur. For those with hypertensive changes (LVH, medial hypertrophy), a TIA or stroke can occur, as blood pressure and blood coagulability change in an uncontrolled manner.

If doctors are to achieve success with CFS and TFE symptoms, they will need to become interested once again in the lives of patients, and not just in their symptoms, signs, and investigation findings. The patient will also need to engage. Patients will need to be encouraged to examine their lives: its successes, failures, and raison d'être. To improve their prognosis, many will need conviction for change: to alter course and prevent further ill-health and medical catastrophe. Half-hearted conviction will not be enough. Some patients will need a complete change of heart and mind, gained through an understanding of just how badly they are progressing in life, and how they 'got it wrong' (energy balance) before getting ill. Only by admitting their mistakes and being ready to learn new strategies will some avoid further illness.

Some patients will need the resolve of David faced with Goliath. How else are they to surmount the obstacles they face? They must come to know, for instance, the part played by their chronic resentment on tiredness, fatigue, and exhaustion, all of which can blind them to the benefits of gratitude, magnanimity, acceptance, tolerance, and forgiveness, when trying to understand their opponents.

Doctors who base their medical practice on technology alone will rarely be interested enough to understand the demise of human beings whose basic components of mind, body, and soul must integrate to form a healthy functioning whole. Those dealing with one-off accident cases, like bone fractures and tumour removal as their primary function, can avoid personal involvement and assume anonymity. Many doctors prefer this, restricting their relationship with patients to a functional level. Conveniently, they may regard anything else as unprofessional, even if in the patient's interest.

The aim of this book is to provide a working framework, model, or hypothesis, to explain TFE and its management, having investigated energy generation at a molecular level, neurotransmission, and integrated cerebral functioning. The result is a clinical framework for understanding and managing CFS and TFE symptoms, that I have found useful in practice.

Using clinical anecdote, epidemiology, electro-encephalography, brain imaging (PET, etc.), the measures necessary to validate the role of energy balance in various medical states in individuals should become better defined.

In Part 1, I consider the clinical features of TFE, its possible molecular and neurobiological origins. I make use of several physical concepts like stress, strain, and constitution, to aid the understanding of individual patient reactions to circumstances and sleep adequacy. Concepts such as resistance, capacitance, and induction, motors, switching and amplification, used in electronic circuits, have biological equivalents that deserve consideration. Also important to clinical practice are two concepts taken from the world of physics: entropy and catastrophe.

In Part 2, I review ancient and modern views of sleep. I consider the role of sleep to conserve and replenish energy and its function in the origin of TFE symptoms. I explore the concept of a life energy equation, and its relationship to ill-health, disease, and medical catastrophe. Based on the model generated, I discuss the management of TFE symptoms.

In Part 3, I have formed conclusions about the origins of TFE symptoms and how a model encompassing energy spending and conservation can help to reduce clinical risk. In the PostScript, I address the practical issues facing doctors who might wish to include clinical energetic principles into their practice. Because the organisation of some clinical practices in the UK is not fit for efficient purpose (Dighton, D.H. 2023), I mention the time and facilities required to assess and treat patients presenting with TFE symptoms.

There are four illustrations. Instead of dispersing the illustrations throughout the text, I have included them in a separate section at the end of the book.

I have examined 'stress' as a threat to homeostasis, and 'strain' in terms of pathophysiological reaction; as biological features, rather than simple physical characteristics. This results in a commonplace concept – the definition of human constitution. My grandmother often referred to it. She would have said that children are born (in late Victorian times) with either a weak or strong constitution. Was she correct? If so, she should have been able to predict individual liability to disease, morbidity, and mortality!

I have defined tiredness, fatigue, and exhaustion, not only as everyday entities, but as significant clinical symptoms. At present, many doctors may prefer to ascribe TFE symptoms to anaemia, diabetes, altered biochemistry or deleterious changes in cardiac or cerebral function, rather than the result of psychosocial factors, poor sleep, and conflict in life.

I have sought answers for the sudden occurrence of medical catastrophe – stroke, cardiac infarction, acute psychosis, pneumonia, septicaemia, and some road traffic accidents. I hope to show that considering human energy as a life equation can contribute to both the understanding of TFE symptoms and the occurrence and progress of many medical conditions.

PART ONE

Chapter One

The Clinical Problem

Mental Tiredness, Fatigue and Exhaustion

I have referred to daytime tiredness as a spectrum increasing from tiredness, through fatigue, to exhaustion as the acronym TFE, rather than referring to diagnostic entities like chronic fatigue syndrome (CFS) or 'vital exhaustion' (VE) with many gained connotations. I have used 'TFE' to represent any perceived state between tiredness and exhaustion, rather than CFS, which specifies fatigue only, or VE that specifies exhaustion only.

Following the First World War, researchers sought a definition and measure of fatigue. The UK formed an Industrial Fatigue (later Health) Research Board in 1921 to serve the purpose. They proposed eliminating "fatigue" from scientific discourse due to its subjectivity and lack of objective verification (Muscio, B. 1921).

Since then, several semi-quantitative questionnaire measures of fatigue have been devised. Among them are the Chronic Illness Fatigue Scale (FACIT-F)(Cella, D. et al. 2010), and the Edmonton Symptom Assessment System (ESAS-r)(Watanabe, S.N. et al. 2012).

In 1950, Hans Selye pioneered the understanding of stress and its clinical effects. He proposed the 'general adaptation syndrome' model. He wrote, 'Anything that causes stress endangers life, unless it is met by adequate adaptive responses; conversely, anything that endangers life causes stress and adaptive responses'.

In describing the immediate and later reactions of the body to emergency situations, he divided responses into three phases:

(1) The Alarm Reaction: a "fight-or-flight" response. The sympathetic nervous system is stimulated, and the body's resources are mobilised to meet the threat.
(2) The Stage of Resistance: The parasympathetic nervous system attempts to return physiological functions to normal.
(3) The Stage of Exhaustion: If the stressor continues beyond the body's extended capacity to cope, resources will seem depleted and strain effects like hypertension, or an increased susceptibility to disease (distress) may become apparent.

He noted that the immediate physiological responses to alarm (parasympathetic, sympathetic, and renin-angiotensin activation, and hormone production, etc.) can disappear during the stage of resistance, and reappear during the stage of exhaustion—a stage where no further physiological adaptation is possible. The 'stage of resistance' is not a clinical phase I have witnessed, since most patients have either an acute or prolonged reaction to stress. Selye made no specific mention of patient 'energy status', and how stress might incite different responses depending on their energy status (TFE). He did, however, suggest response polymorphism—the same stress producing various responses in different individuals.

Human beings, going about their everyday business, will function on the energy spectrum, somewhere from 'full of energy' to exhaustion, with tiredness and fatigue observed between the extremes. Tiredness is a subjective symptom, the natural result of human physical and mental activity. No human who has experienced a lack of energy will deny that it can be slight (tiredness), inhibiting (fatigue), or extreme and disabling (exhaustion). In different cultures, different words will describe these perceptions, some with overlapping nuances.

The topic of addressing the individual use of energy is complex. We all need to learn how our free-ranging human activity relates to the energy we have, but many make mistakes. Like all other subjective assessments (beauty, common sense, happiness, and acceptable behaviour), the relevance and significance of some information is a matter of individual judgment. As with all forms of art, all attempts at standardisation will fail; remaining never more than a bureaucratic aspiration. Many have attempted to assess human circumstances, relationships, life change, personality, and behaviour using questionnaires. In everyday life, however, its dependable assessment remains an art form.

The objective model used in science—defining, categorising, and selecting compliant data for analysis is only partially applicable to subjective symptoms, like those of TFE. This is not, however, a valid argument for dismissing human energy and its apparent depletion, as meaningless concepts; one of the commonest of all human complaints, found more in female patients (20.4%) than in males (14.3%) (Chen, M. 1986). Studies of human energy remain descriptive, and at best (from an inappropriate scientific viewpoint), measurable only in semi-quantitative terms with questionnaires, reaction time tests, and behavioural reactions. Despite their lack of independent validity, these methods can reveal aspects of human energy exchange that are essential for normal human functioning.

TFE symptoms are common to many medical conditions. They include psychiatric disorders, post-viral and other recovery states. When a satisfactory explanation is lacking, one can always make a default diagnosis of Chronic Fatigue Syndrome. Many cases will involve entities that lie beyond standard medical intervention, like aging, athleticism, social circumstances, and motivation. Their contribution needs to be considered, using a common framework that accounts for energy turnover; energy spending and repletion.

To be useful clinically, the measurement of TFE symptoms would measure cerebral energy storage, utilisation, and turnover in relation to neurotransmitter and EEG activity. Despite the use of various imaging techniques for this purpose, none has yet achieved scientific holy grail status.

Until that happens, I have defined the individual TFE symptoms as:

- Tiredness is that mental state perceived as a mild lack of energy. One can overcome it by necessity, motivation, novel stimulation, or one night of restful sleep.

- Fatigue is that further state of tiredness, recognised by a lack of perceived energy and an inability to perform more, once given adequate motivation or stimulus.

- Exhaustion is a state of extreme tiredness (a feeling of energy depletion) characterised by a complete inability to perform, whatever the strength of motivating stimuli. If required to perform, performance could deteriorate, become unstable or lead to catastrophe.

Normal human functioning performance (cognitive tasks, etc.) is often proportional to need, or the strength of motivation. Subjectively, it also relates to the perceived energy available. It follows a simple model, based on the everyday observation of human activity (Fig. 1)(Nixon, P.G. 1976).

With increasing arousal, necessity will boost the energy we experience, and work can proceed without fatigue. In the longer term, multiple responses to stimulation (lasting many minutes or hours), will cause tiring. Further stimulation might produce more work, but with less efficiency and more mistakes. At this point, the individual is fatigued. Perceived as a low energy state, further demand results in little more work accomplished. When subjects are exhausted, any stimulation results in either no work or the deterioration of work results. Exhaustion can precede collapse, be it physical or mental. In a state of collapse, the subject is completely incapacitated and unable to act further. At this stage, many types of catastrophic change can occur: failure to cope – commonly referred to as a 'mental breakdown' – accidents while driving, or the onset of cardiac infarction or stroke. Even with every risk factor accounted for, responses are hard to predict.

My colleague Dr. Peter Nixon published the normal human stimulus / performance characteristics as 'The Human Function Curve' (Fig. 1) in 1976, while we were both working at Charing Cross Hospital, London. In the current work, I have extended the concept by exploring the molecular and neurophysiological basis for TFE symptoms, and how they might relate to cardiovascular disease and its control.

The model illustrated in Fig. 1, was partly based on Dr. Peter Nixon's army experience of training soldiers. They had to withstand extreme motivational arousal for acceptance into an élite fighting unit. The 'Human Function Curve' only reflects the relationship between performance (p) and arousal (A)(the pA relationship) in normal people at one time. I added bi-stability and catastrophic change, to account for sudden cardiac infarction (once arterial disease has developed 90% stenosis), or cerebral haemorrhage secondary to hypertension.

The level of tiredness experienced by subjects will change their pA relationship. Several life function curves are therefore necessary to reflect functioning during different TFE states (Fig. 2). The latter model has proven valuable for understanding the clinical functioning of patients with TFE symptoms. The greater the degree of TFE, the more difficult it may be to control diabetes, psoriasis, infection, blood pressure, or coagulability.

Peter Nixon later wrote: 'The paradigm (the human function curve) accommodates catastrophe theory and provides an unambiguous basis for screening and intervention in hypertension and coronary heart disease where there is a self-defeating struggle to close the ever-widening gap between the actual performance capability and the intended.' (Nixon, P.G. 1982).

The Status of TFE Symptoms

With under-stimulation, in low-demand environments (on holiday), low arousal can cause sleepiness, lassitude, sloth, and a lack of energy for task completion. Both a sleep deficit and a relaxing environment can induce it. In the absence of work demands, natural sleep patterns readily emerge, and the post-prandial energy dip after lunch can lead to a nap or siesta. Some work schedules can overcome the pressure to sleep. There would seem to be two forms of simple tiredness: that which follows repeated stimulation, and that associated with under-stimulation. Imprisonment can cause a mixture of both. With intolerable environmental conditions, insomnia, and daytime tiredness are common (Dewa, L.H. et al. 2017).

Tiredness is a subjective state, readily induced by repetitive, uninteresting work, and relieved by novelty or the prospect of enjoyment. It can get worse without future prospects and no immediate likelihood of change. People may exhibit avoidance behaviour, especially when life feels overwhelming or beyond their capabilities. It can attract help from those more capable.

The connotations of TFE symptoms are usually social or medical. Although TFE symptoms are non-specific, they can be the first sign of specific illness or disease, or signal declining general or mental health.

Fatigue has emotional, behavioural, and cognitive components, whose inter-relationships are mostly unexplored (Lewis, G. 1992). Also unexplored are the neurobiology, neuro-pathophysiology and molecular aspects of TFE symptoms.

Some degree of TFE is common in everyday life. One Scandinavian survey showed fatigue occurring twice as frequently as exhaustion (Tibblin, G, et al. 1990). In my own unpublished survey of over one thousand cases, all of whom were complaining of TFE symptoms, only 5% had physical disease (after multiple screening investigations). Many had high anxiety, depression, and obsession scores on a Middlesex Hospital (Neuroticism) Questionnaire (MHQ). A few, had raised Ebstein-Barr (EB) antibodies (IgG and IgM), suggesting the possibility of EB virus infection as a cause, although its ubiquity in many western countries is a consideration. My investigations did not include EB antigen as an indicator of active infection.

TFE is common and often engages GP services in the UK. Its prevalence makes it a significant medical management challenge.

TFE most commonly presents as excessive daytime sleepiness associated with defective sleep at night. The exceptions are clinical conditions with TFE as a common symptom (hypothyroidism, Addison's disease, various infectious diseases, dementia, depression, etc.). In the absence of an obvious clinical cause, it can present with various associations: as depression, demoralisation, lack of motivation, or poor BP and diabetic control. Fatigue and exhaustion are associated with significant risks: of road traffic accidents, cardiac infarction, acute psychosis, stroke, and worsening or more difficult to control, psoriasis or infection, etc. TFE symptoms thus deserve to be recognised as a clue to underlying disease, a disease modifier, or the result of stresses affecting sleep quality.

TFE: Assumptions and Postulates

Before any further enquiry, an examination of the assumptions held, and the postulates accepted about human energy, is essential. The following need consideration:

- Energy is neither created nor destroyed, only transferred.
- All mental and physical work requires a power supply.
- Dietary nutrients supply the substrate for ATP production – the primary source of cellular energy.
- All perceived human energy (physical and mental) comes

from intracellular, mitochondrial ATP synthesis.

- Astrocyte synthesis of ATP is blood glucose and glycogenolysis dependent. The availability of the lactate produced as an energy source is transporter dependent (monocarboxylate transporter). Astrocyte glycogen is reduced during wakefulness and repleted by sleep.

- Exhausting physical exercise reduces both astrocyte and muscle glycogen. Physical exhaustion depletes muscle glycogen and the mental component of endurance depletes astrocyte glycogen (Matsui, T. et al. 2017).

- For evolutionary and survival purposes, the availability of ATP for healthy functioning, can be regarded as infinite. ATP synthesis can be reduced by mitochondrial disease (mutations in both nuclear DNA (nDNA) and mitochondrial DNA (mtDNA); during mitochondrial flashes, and by the negative feedback loop involving phosphofructokinase-1 (PFK1) and pyruvate kinase).(Shepherd, R.K. et al. 2006)(Dunn, J. & Grider, M.H. 2023).

- Any failure to synthesise ATP will lead to disease or death.

- Whether ATP synthesis (producing half to one human bodyweight of ATP each day), is defective in those who experience TFE is unknown.

Life is possible only by converting chemical energy into:

- Electrical energy (ionic flux): Na+ influx driven action potentials, when integrated in different areas of the brain, underlies consciousness, thinking, emotion and all mental processing.

- Mechanical energy that allows the work of skeletal muscle, and smooth muscle in genito-urinary, and gastrointestinal systems, together with cardiac muscle (not the subject of this treatise).

ATP is required for both.

- Only one gram (approximately) of the 45 – 70 Kgs of ATP synthesised daily is stored.

- The longer term repositories of cellular biological energy are glycogen and fat. TFE symptoms are not related to their depletion. The only connection relates to the delivery of glucose to neurones by an adequate arterial circulation. TFE will occur if a diminished blood supply reduces the delivery of glucose to neurones (during vasomotor syncope or from cerebral artery disease).

- With TFE symptoms, the lack of capacity to increase cognitive functioning relates to increased cerebral activity in some areas of the brain, and reduced activity in others, with little reserve available for improved functioning (Bremner, J.D. 2004).

- TFE symptoms are not yet understood in cellular neuro-biological, energetic terms.

- TFE symptoms relate to the perception of reduced energy available (mental and physical) for completing tasks.

- TFE symptoms are common.

- TFE symptoms affect otherwise healthy people and patients with medical conditions.

- TFE symptoms are associated with an adverse effect on quality of life and work productivity.

- Many diseases present with TFE symptoms initially, and can deteriorate progressively throughout the course of a disease. This raises important clinical questions:

To what extent can the presence of TFE symptoms predict disease?

How might the presence of TFE symptoms affect prognosis?

Measuring TFE

The prevalence of fatigue has been assessed. One survey, using a mailed questionnaire to Norwegians, found 11.4% with substantial fatigue lasting over six months. More women than men complained. Fatigue, age or other social variables showed no relationship. Those with disabilities and psychiatric problems complained more (Loge, J.H. et al. 1998).

Attempts have been made to measure fatigue. Semi-quantitative, psychometric questionnaires allow for the reproducible measurement of fatigue. The Multidimensional Fatigue Inventory, with twenty questions, provides a reliable measure of general fatigue, physical fatigue, mental fatigue, reduced motivation and reduced activity. Smets, E.M. et al. (1995), found it reliable for cancer patients receiving radiotherapy and those diagnosed with chronic fatigue syndrome. Others have used the Fatigue Assessment Scale (Michielsen, H. J., et al. 1998), and the Fatigue Symptom Inventory (Hann, D. M., et al. 1998).

To find the non-disease related causes of fatigue, De Rijk, A. E., et al., examined the antecedent factors for the patient complaint: 'I'm so tired!' They used the Multidimensional Fatigue Inventory (MFI-20) to assess external stimulation. They found overload (quantity of stimulation) to be related to general and mental fatigue. When assessing the quality of stimulation, an unattractive background to the stimulation was associated with high fatigue scores; a background perceived as 'attractive', resulted in lower scores. Both the quantity and quality of external stimulation were thus assessed (the Quality–Quantity model for understanding fatigue). They also found that depression, measured using a questionnaire, 'directly and strongly related to all dimensions of fatigue'.

Clinical Energy Considerations

The Greek word 'enirgeia', meaning work, gave rise to the word 'energy'. Energetics is the science or study of energy, first used in the late 19th century in relation to animals.

'There is energy due to motion called kinetic energy, energy due to gravitational interaction (gravitational potential energy, it is called), thermal energy, electrical energy, light energy, elastic energy in springs and so on, chemical energy, nuclear energy - and there is also an energy that a particle has from its mere existence, an energy that depends directly on its mass. The last is the contribution of Einstein, as you undoubtedly know. $E=mc^2$ is the famous equation of the law I am talking about.'

Richard P. Feynman. The Character of Physical Law.

In the beginning, there was energy. The creation of the universe required it, so did we. We can neither make energy nor destroy it, but we can store it and use it to build a life of our own making (overcoming entropy). Energy can create new structures (increasing entropy) or to destroy them (decreasing entropy). No other options exist other than acquiring it, using, or storing it. An awareness of these choices, and how to use them, can make the difference between our personal failure and success, our health, and ill-health, and sometimes life or death.

The second law of thermodynamics indicates that the organisation of the universe will gradually decay until all particles are evenly distributed throughout. This homogeny represents a low energy state with no structure (low entropy). To build a living creature requires lots of energy to create functional structure. Maintaining the structures necessary for life (homeostasis) requires energy to overcome the natural process of disintegration. Healthy humans can manage this for 80-years. What has developed over evolutionary time is a biological, chemical factory capable of converting hydrogen, carbon, oxygen, phosphorus, sodium, potassium, magnesium, nitrogen (etc.) into cells powered by the high-energy phosphate bonds of ATP. ATP represents locked-in energy, available to power homeostasis.

At a personal level, the energy we have is a fundamental resource. Without it, humans can neither survive nor achieve success by endeavour. Without it, we cannot empower our talent and intelligence to plan and execute the life we want to lead. We use energy to power our ego as a driving force, and to comply with the social mores of friends, family, and our adopted culture. Energy is required for the constant adaptation required for social compatibility. Without sufficient energy available, our mind, body, and preferred social order will disintegrate.

The medical significance of TFE symptoms is not always appreciated. As part of a full clinical examination and investigation, one should question its origins: the nature of the person (anxious, depressed, obsessional, Type A personality); social circumstances (stressors at home and work), and quality of sleep, especially if they have established hypertension or coronary artery disease (CHD). Instead of addressing TFE symptoms—a once fundamental role for every medical practitioner (Hippocratic medicine)—specialised doctors may ignore these inquiries or refer patients to counsellors, psychiatrists, social workers, or alternative therapists.

The presence of TFE symptoms has associations that affect quality of life, risking:

- Failure of motivation.
- Failure to enjoy life.
- Failure to cope with life problems.
- Failure to achieve self-esteem through success.
- Failure of health.

I have observed an occasional association with resistant hypertension and worsening angina. These conditions can be improved by sleep, taking holidays, yoga and other methodologies aimed at diffusing anxiety, worry, fear, panic, over-reaction, overactivity and stress. As a consequence, I have seen hypertension more easily controlled, and the walking distance of those with angina, improved. Unfortunately, the results are inconsistent, because psychological and physical responses to comparable stressors are variable.

The presence of TFE symptoms can exacerbate clinical symptoms, if not the pathological process involved. Clearly, the severity and rapidity of some disease processes, can override all other considerations. With chronic conditions, the patient's history can indicate a susceptibility to stress, TFE, and sleep disturbance. When difficulty is found controlling symptoms, blood pressure, diabetes, or infection, attributing significance to TFE can prove worthwhile.

The role TFE might play in the aetiology of disease is unclear. Its role in the progress of disease is better documented—the more severe the TFE, the more it is likely to enhance progress. Epidemiological studies suggest its validity as a predictive factor (see the following section).

As an example, clinicians need to know when the disquiet and disturbed sleep of bereavement might increase the risk of pneumonia, cardiac infarction, stroke, or cancer? Clinicians sometimes observe such connections.

TFE: Epidemiology and Associated Medical Conditions

The origins of fatigue in the workplace, relate to the perception of work-stress, organizational support, supervisor support, and staff health, modified by psychological stress, anxiety, and depression. The origins of fatigue also relate to expected work outcomes, turnover, organizational commitment, and job satisfaction (Pawlikowska, T. 1994).

How does fatigue relate to illness? It is not surprising to find that some women awaiting chemotherapy for breast cancer, have stressful concerns that lead to fatigue. In a group of such patients, fatigue was found associated with sleep disturbance and circadian rhythm delay. Although their circadian rhythm mostly remained robust, those with delayed rhythms experienced more daily dysfunction (Ancoli-Israel, S. et al. 2006).

'Vital exhaustion' has been found associated with cardiovascular disease (CVD)(Frestad, D. 2017), the metabolic syndrome (Pedersen, J. et al 2016), chronic obstructive pulmonary disease (Clark, A. et al.), weight gain, the risk of obesity (Iversen, L. et al. 2012), and all-cause mortality.

TFE symptoms and depression can overlap, but can be differentiated (Balog, P. et al. 2017)(Kop, W. 2012)(van Dienst, R. 1991). TFE symptoms can be reduced when selective serotonin reuptake inhibitors (SSRIs) are prescribed.

In those with COPD, tiredness, walking distance, and depression are associated (Breslin, E., et al., 1998). TFE is a common clinical feature of infectious and chronic inflammatory disease, heart failure, advanced cancer, stroke, uncontrolled diabetes, and anaemia (more often causing shortness of breath than TFE at rest).

Can TFE warn of catastrophe? To test the hypothesis that TFE symptoms might predict myocardial infarction, Appels, A. et al. (1988), followed 3877 males with known ischaemic heart disease for 4.2 years (aged 39-65 years). Of the 59 who sustained a myocardial infarction (MI), preceding feelings of exhaustion appeared predictive on multiple logistic regression analysis (having controlled for smoking, age, BP, blood cholesterol, and medication). Appels (Appels, A., Falger, P.R. 1993) further showed that similar results also apply to women. The presence of 'vital exhaustion' was found to be 2.75 times more common in pre-infarction women, than in those hospitalised for orthopaedic problems. Patients with 'vital exhaustion' (VE)(Maastricht Questionnaire; Shahid, A., et al. 2011) who developed unusual fatigue, irritability, and dejection, were more likely to develop angina (RR: 1.86), and non-fatal infarction (RR: 2.28). VE and fatal events were not found linked.

The presence of fatigue can predict secondary events following angioplasty (Kop, W.J. et al. 1994). They followed a group of post-angioplasty patients (n=127) for an average of 1.5 years. During that time, fifteen of the 43 exhausted patients (35%), developed a new cardiac event. Only 14 of the 84 (17%), who were not exhausted, experienced a new cardiac event (RR: 2.7). Among the new events were cardiac death, myocardial infarction, coronary bypass surgery, repeat-PTCA, increase of coronary atherosclerosis, or new anginal complaints with documented ischaemia.

Vital exhaustion has been found as a primary risk factor for both cardiac infarction (doubling the risk)(Schuitemaker, G.E., et al. 2004) and first stroke (Schuitemaker, G.E., 2004).

CHAPTER TWO

Neurobiological Energetics and TFE Symptoms

The following are presumed to be accepted assumptions and postulates:

- All humans need sleep; enough to allow efficient daytime functioning.

- Without restorative sleep, humans suffer TFE in various degrees, both in the long and short term.

- Arousal progresses from deep unconsciousness, through reflexive responsiveness, to full waking consciousness and intellectual capacity.

- There are stages of arousal from deeply unconscious, through to having reactive reflexes only, to being awake, wilful and fully capable intellectually.

- To function at all, the brain has basal physiological requirements: a blood flow at sufficient arterial pressure (> 60mms Hg); enough glucose and oxygen, together with no excess of CO2.

- A lack of arterial pressure (< 60mms Hg), diminished arterial oxygen saturation (PaO2 < 10kPa), increased CO2, > PaCO2 >5.6kPa (MedlinePlus: blood gases), and glucose (<2.3–2.7 mmol/l [41–49 mg/dl]. Cryer, P.E. 2007) can cause unconsciousness and brain death.

- Astrocyte glycogen storage is decreased with daytime activity and is restored during sleep (Öz, G. et al. 2007)

- Sedative drugs can cause relaxation and unconsciousness.

- The sleeping (and unconscious) brain generates slow voltage waves (0.5 to 7 cycles/second [cps]). EEGs arise from the integration of all neuronal depolarisations.

- The conscious brain generates voltage waves (> 6 to 31cps), with the resultant of integrated depolarisations recorded as EEGs.

- The amplitude of EEG voltage waves varies from 10 to 100 microvolts.

- In 'disturbed' sleep (as reported by patients), there is less slow-wave sleep (low energy dissipation) and more REM sleep (high-energy dissipation sleep).

- Brain power dissipation (P) can be calculated as $P \square 2\pi fA$, where 'f' is frequency and 'A' is amplitude. The higher the level of consciousness, the greater the power expressed by EEGs.

- Slow wave sleep requires minimal power dissipation; solving conscious problems (and REM processing) require maximal power dissipation.

- Cell membrane electrical repolarisation requires the generation of googol numbers of high-energy molecules (ATP) per second.

- Effective sleep, relaxing behaviour (low-load, fast mental functioning – that which requires little cognitive or emotional processing) – and physical activity, reduce mental energy expenditure.

- In the short term (1-2 days), subjective feelings of tiredness are usually restored by 'effective' sleep.

- Relaxing behaviours (massage, yoga, meditation, enjoyable events, and environments) and distractions (like some sports, playing a musical instrument, etc.), will minimise brain energy expenditure and the need for ATP synthesis.

- 'Defective sleep' is ineffective in reversing TFE and may advance it (from tiredness through to exhaustion).

- Chronic TFE is not reversed by a single night of restful sleep.

- Reversing chronic TFE symptoms (chronic fatigue syndrome), requires a mental workload reduction (solving the longer-term, stressful problems that caused it), together with repeated episodes of effective sleep and continuing daytime relaxation (low-load, fast mental functioning only, requiring little cognitive or emotional processing.

Some questions arise:

- What is 'effective' and 'defective' sleep?

- Does short-term mental energy deprivation (TFE symptoms) differ neurophysiologically and biochemically from that occurring in the longer term?

- Does the tiredness associated with inactivity and relaxation differ from that resulting from increased mental activity?

- What cerebral molecular changes occur in relation to TFE and its reversal? Can decreased ATP synthesis and increased ATP utilisation cause TFE symptoms?

- How much chemical energy is stored at any one time?

- Can total brain power and energy utilisation be measured?

- In refreshing sleep, are neuronal pathways re-set (unblocked or inhibition removed)?

- Does sleep restore energy and neuro-transmitter stores?

Clinicians valued rest, relaxation, sleep, recuperation, and convalescence well before the era of 'scientific medicine'. For ancient Greeks, sleep was a time when Æsculapius visited their mind and did healing work. To maintain the fitness of their soldiers, the Spartans used the cycle: fight, sleep, train physically, and fight again.

Cerebral Electrical and Molecular Activity Data from Neuro-imaging

Brain imaging has been undertaken in those with obsession-compulsion disorder (OCD), phobia, post-traumatic stress disorder PTSD, fear, anxiety, and panic. These results are of interest because these conditions can generate TFE symptoms.

Neuroimaging techniques include positron emission (PET), single photon emission (SPECT) and MRI, functional MRI (fMRI) and MRI spectroscopy. The detection of N-acetyl aspartate (NAA) can be used as a marker of neuronal integrity; metabolism can be measured using radioactive glucose fluoro-deoxyglucose (FDG).

NMR spectroscopy has been used to measure glycogen content and turnover in the brain of human volunteers. Glucose 1-(13)C was infused for durations up to fifty hours, and brain glycogen labelling and washout were measured in the occipital lobe for up to 84 hours. Human brain glycogen content was estimated at approximately 3.5 micromols/g. (three to fourfold higher than free glucose at euglycemia). 'Turnover of bulk brain glycogen occurred at a rate of 0.16 micromols per gram per hour, implying that complete turnover requires 3-5 days. Twenty minutes of visual stimulation did not result in detectable glycogen utilization in the visual cortex, as judged from similar [13C] glycogen levels before and after stimulation. We conclude that the brain stores a substantial amount of glycogen relative to free glucose and metabolises this store very slowly under normal physiology.' (Öz, G., et al. 2007). The same group estimated the brain content of glycogen to be 7.8 ± 0.3 µmol/g. (Öz, G., et al. 2015).

With anxiety and obsessional-compulsive disorder (OCD) as clinical features, Bremner, J.D. (2004), found evidence of changes in brain blood flow, metabolism, and tissue volume. These he observed in the hippocampus, amygdala, cingulate, prefrontal and parietal cortex. The changes were in either a positive or negative direction, depending on the brain location and clinical condition.

In PTSD, there are areas that increase or decrease brain tissue blood flow and volume (a decrease being associated with defective short-term memory). Stress can interfere with hippocampal function, including long-term memory potentiation. The mechanisms proposed include elevated levels of glucocorticoids (during stress), stress-related inhibition of brain-derived neurotrophic factor, changes in serotonergic function, and inhibition of neurogenesis in the hippocampus. In isolated neuronal cell preparations, glucocorticoids can speed the decline of cellular ATP concentrations during metabolic insults like aglycaemia (Lawrence and Sapolsky. 1994). This finding cannot be extrapolated to global cerebral functioning without making many assumptions. As a related observation, I saw glucocorticoids remove fatigue and activate mental processes in a case of Addison's disease. The patient claimed 'to have gained control over his energy' by adjusting his cortisol treatment doses.

In social phobic disorder, functional imaging studies can detect increased activity in the amygdala and hippocampus. In OCD, imaging studies have detected dysfunction in the frontal lobe, in a striatal–orbito-frontal circuit, as well as dysfunction in the striatum for ritualistic behaviour.

Neuroimaging studies have confirmed that the brain areas involved in stress, memory and emotion also play a role in anxiety disorders. A close link exists between anxiety disorder and stress. A smaller hippocampal volume and/or reduced markers of neuronal integrity (N-acetyl aspartate) have been found in PTSD. Other anxiety disorders have not been associated with smaller hippocampal volume. Other corroborative evidence exists (Diamond, D.M., et al. 1996; Gurvits, T.G., et al. 1996); Bremner. J.D., et al. 1999; Breiter, H.C., et al. 1996).

Sleep deprivation is common in stressed subjects with TFE symptoms. Patients cannot sleep well, and feel they have not been 're-charged' by (disturbed) sleep. Wu, J.C., et al. (1991), reported the effect of total sleep deprivation (about 32-hour) on human subjects, on regional cerebral glucose metabolism during wakefulness. They used positron emission tomography (PET), with F-18 deoxyglucose (FDG). They concluded that: 'Sleep deprivation leads to a significant reorganization of regional cerebral metabolic activity, with relative decreases in the temporal lobes and increases in visual cortex. Absolute glucose metabolic measurements indicate a decrease in thalamus, basal ganglia, white matter, and cerebellum. No overall decrease in whole brain metabolism was noted after sleep deprivation. As expected, sleep deprivation significantly reduced visual vigilance as assessed by the continuous performance test and this decrease was correlated significantly with reduced metabolic rate in thalamic, basal ganglia, and limbic regions.'

The TFE symptoms caused by sleep deprivation can be associated with focal cerebral metabolic changes. Mental fatigue might exert demands on the neural processes necessary for efficient information processing (Cook, D.B., et al. 2007). They showed: 'Brain regions that were significantly related to mental fatigue included the parietal, cingulate, inferior frontal and superior temporal cortices, cerebellum and cerebellar vermis; regions that have been demonstrated as important for several aspects of cognitive function, including those that involve the working memory network.' Their brain MRI results showed human mental fatigue related to brain activity when subjects undertook a mentally fatiguing cognitive task. Exaggerated neural responses in several regions of the brain were associated with chronic fatigue.

In global cerebral terms, fatigue is associated with both increases and decreases in the focal neuronal activity of different regions. It is also associated with the interruption of neuronal activity in Alzheimer dementia and in multiple sclerosis.

Brain Power and EEG Waveforms

In 1875, Richard Caton made the first known animal recordings of brain activity. In 1924, Hans Berger, a German psychiatrist, pioneered the use of EEG in humans.

An EEG detects the resultant of all neuronal and axonal action potential ionic activity, thought generated by cortical pyramidal neurones. The power (P) represented by any EEG waveform is proportional to its frequency ('f') and amplitude ('A'): $P \square 2\pi fA$.

EEG voltage waveforms must traverse the brain, CSF, meninges, and the skull before being detected. The result will suffer interference from other electrical activity, like the ECG. EEGs result from differential amplification, recording voltage differences between pairs of electrodes. (Britton, J.W. et al. 2016). The global, cerebral ionic activity, that produces the EEG, represents the resultant of integrated wave fronts, created by out-of-phase neuronal depolarisation in different areas. Waves will sometimes combine to get augmented. Others will nullify. Like ECGs, EEG voltages are subject to vector considerations, varying in strength with direction and dependent on recording electrode positioning.

Like ECGs, EEG voltages are subject to vector considerations, varying in strength with direction and dependent on recording electrode positioning.

Frequency is used to classify EEG waves. Many changes are seen accompanying wakeful cerebral activity and different phases of sleep, and through several levels of unconsciousness induced by anaesthesia.

Mental Effort and the EEG

Mental activity consumes power. The biochemical functioning of neurones, the production of neurotransmitters, ATP synthesis, the maintenance of a negative cellular potential, the transmission of depolarisation down axons and the restoration of the intracellular negative potential afterwards, all require power.

Two important questions arise:

- What is the relationship between the EEG (using its amplitude and frequency) and the actually energy used for brain activity?
- Can an EEG reflect the energy dynamics responsible for TFE symptoms?

EEG brainwave function changes with increasing cognitive workload (Fitzgibbon, S.P. et al. 2004). This has been investigated in various ways. Some researchers have measured EEG spectral power (displaying a function of frequency and amplitude), and evoked responses (Brouwer, A.M. et al. 2012) (Zhu, Y., et al. 2021).

Increased task difficulty (scientific problem solving) yielded higher frontal theta power and lower parieto-occipital alpha power.

During tasks similar to those needed for air traffic control (for two hours), the spectral power of five different EEG recording sites increased with time on task (Desari, D. et al. 2017). Recorded EEGs, were associated with several cerebral functions: visual perception, cognitive processing, and motor outputs. They concluded that: 'different levels of mental factors can be sensitively reflected in EEG signals associated with various brain functions, including real-world tasks.'

With more sub-tasks performed, theta activity in the frontal region increases and alpha activity of the parietal region decreases. (Puma, S. et al. 2018). Holm, A. et al (2009), used a wearable, 2-channel EEG device to measure the theta Fz/alpha Pz ratio as a calculated index (Fz = midline frontal recording; Pz = midline parietal recording). They concluded: 'The index increased with the number of tasks to be performed concurrently ($p = 0.004$) and with increased time awake, both after normal sleep ($p = 0.002$) and sleep restriction ($p = 0.004$). Moreover, the increase of the index was more pronounced in the afternoon after sleep restriction ($p = 0.006$). As a measure of brain state and its dynamics, the index can be considered equivalent to the heartbeat, an indicator of the cardiovascular state, thus inspiring the name "brainbeat".'

Using EEGs, one can monitor the state of unconsciousness in anaesthesia (Kim, M. C. et al. 2020; preferably using their spectral analysis. The changes seen depend on anaesthetic dose. As anaesthesia progresses, the oscillatory spectral power of fast waves decreases, and the power of slow waves increases. Alpha and delta slow wave power increases with short periods of electrical inactivity. Theta waves can become dominant in the frontal areas.

Computed oscillatory power spectra (frequency and power in dBs), reveal distinct changes with different anaesthetics. Sevoflurane anaesthesia increases theta and beta oscillation power. Its binding to glutamate binding sites on NMDA and non-NMDA receptors may cause the changes seen with ketamine. These block excitatory pathways. Ketamine also binds to cholinergic, opioid, and monoamine receptors. During ketamine anaesthesia, gamma bursts may reflect this inhibition. Increased theta and gamma oscillation power and decreased alpha / beta oscillatory power follows them.

There is much speculation about the mechanisms that serve EEG generation. For instance, researchers have associated increased alpha waves with GABAa decay (time and conductance), and delta waves with the 'on' and 'off' states of neurones. Because EEG waves vary with age, some suggest that ionic currents, myelin integrity, and synaptic density are all involved in the generation of EEG oscillatory power spectra.

Brain Power

In Fig 3., the schematic provides a conception of brain power from minimal to maximal. Escalating energy demands accompany the brain's shifting consciousness, ranging from deep unconsciousness to full alertness. The key steps are these:

- In its basal state, the unconscious brain produces very little EEG activity, but some energy is required for basic neuronal cell, brainstem functioning. The continuance of normal, vital brainstem functioning is essential if life is to continue. This is guaranteed by efficient energy supply mechanisms: a sufficient blood supply (hence, the Circle of Willis); a constant supply of O2, the constant removal of CO2, and an almost infinite supply of glucose, ATP, and neurotransmitters.

- Slow wave sleep activity (SWS) during NREM sleep adds another level of energy requirement.

- REM sleep and subconscious processing, consumes yet more energy, albeit intermittently.

- Arousal and consciousness occur first in a non-thinking, non-emotive, tranquil state. Energy is required to maintain this level of consciousness.

- Increasing levels of cognitive and emotional processing vary from simple, fast, start to finish transactions (fast thinking [Kahneman, D. 2011]), like deciding to get out of bed, to the complicated processing (slow thinking) required for evaluation, judgment, and decision making.

- Long-term cognitive, interactional and emotional solving (slow thinking), with no easy, immediate solution, can make the brain refractory to solving other problems. A continuing concern about such problems needs a constant energy supply. Heightened REM sleep may be associated. Could the extra power dissipated be responsible for the feeling of being stressed and overburdened? Clinically progressive TFE symptoms are likely to arise without power reduction measures.

- Energy expenditure (E) follows a 24-hour cycle, while the following integral represents total power (P) consumption from time t1 to t2:

$$P = \int E.dt. (t1 - t2)$$

The EEG spectral oscillatory power (in time), calculated from the wave frequency and amplitude, will increase from basal functioning (in a vegetative state), to slow wave sleep, and then to a high-functioning cognitive state (Fig 3).

If we could measure total brain power, would it relate to TFE status? This is unlikely, given that specific pathways alone may be required for the perception of limited mental energy. Since the brain has no definable 'battery' storage area, power calculations using EEGs are unlikely to reflect TFE symptoms.

Energy Considerations and Neuronal Electrical Activity

Roy and Sherringham, in 1890, proposed a link between neuronal activity, cerebral blood flow, energy use, and metabolic alterations. We now know that 55.6% of those with small vessel cerebral artery disease have associated fatigue (Jolly, A.A., et al. 2014).

Maintaining the intracellular/extracellular voltage difference (using the $Na+/K+$ pump for the ion gradient) requires energy for the electrical steady state of every neuronal cell. The hydrolysis of ATP to ADP (and AMP) produces this energy. The depolarisation of cells required for the neuronal activity that underlies mental work first involves the activation of $Na+$ channels. Sodium enters the cell to initiate depolarisation, while potassium escapes. The $Na+/K+$ pump will spend much energy restoring the ion gradient and potential difference. The depolarisation wave then propagates down an axon until it meets a synapse. At this point, it induces further transmission by inciting the release of neurotransmitter(s).

Regulatory processes exist for cellular ATP production. 'Ca2+ acts through multiple pathways to increase ATP synthesis, matching energy supply to demand. Increasing cytosolic Ca2+ stimulates metabolite transfer across the inner mitochondrial membrane through activation of Ca2+ regulated mitochondrial carriers, while an increase in matrix Ca2+ stimulates the citric acid cycle and the ATP synthase'. (Llorente-Folch, I., 2015).

Depolarisation can be incited by acetylcholine (ACh), ATP, and other transmitters co-stored in presynaptic vesicles. All cerebral activity is therefore dependent on the manufacture of ACh, ATP, and other transmitters.

If neurotransmitter and ATP production (among other compounds) provide power for brain activity, how much energy must the brain produce and use per second? How might these factors change with TFE? No objective answer exists for the second question. The best information available relates the energy used by the brain to either O2 consumption, or brain power calculated from EEG activity.

The oxygen consumption in rabbit brains is cerebral blood flow dependent (Fujita, N. 1956). Although the brain amounts to only 2% of bodyweight, it consumes 20% of the oxygen and 25% of the glucose available. Neuronal activity consumes 75% of brain energy.

The brain utilises energy at the synapse, with a large proportion spent restoring neuronal membrane potentials after depolarization (Harris, J.J. et al. 2012). The brain's energy requirements are not uniform; they are increased in the areas of most neuronal activity (Watts, M.E., et al. 2018).

Disruption of oxygen metabolism and mitochondrial function occurs in various age-related neurodegenerative diseases associated with cognitive decline (Tabrizi, S.J. et al. 2000)(Silverman, D.H. et al. 2001). Mitochondrial function is linked to aging by mitochondrial DNA (mtDNA) haplotypes.

Blood-oxygen-level dependent (BOLD), fMRI scanning, has been used to measure brain O2 utilisation (van Zijl, P.C. et al. 2012). It follows neuronal activity. Neuronal function is sensitive to hypoxia. In the adult brain, hypoxia can trigger gene expression, increased neuronal stem cell proliferation and neurogenesis. Reactive oxygen species (ROS) can cause cellular damage through oxidation of lipids, proteins, and DNA. Significant increases in this activity are associated with amyloid plaque formation and dementia.

'To compensate for varying energy demands throughout the brain, and to increase efficiency of metabolite supply, neurovascular and neurometabolic coupling mechanisms have evolved to enhance blood flow and utilization of metabolites in areas of neural activity'. (Watts, M.E., et al. 2018). Neuronal metabolism depends on localised blood flow, partly controlled by neuronal nitric oxide (NO) production and Ca2+ signalling. Improving the supply of oxygen and glucose to the brain will depend on blood supply (in the brain, blood pressure dependent).

ATP Production, and Usage

The production of ATP is remarkable, involving the rotary mechanism of ATP synthase (Nakamoto, R.K. et al. 2008). This was first suggested by Boyer in 1989, who hypothesised that rotation of one or more molecular subunits was an intrinsic part of the catalytic mechanism. ATP synthase is a large complex of at least 22 subunits. The rotary movement of these subunits plays an essential role in both transport and catalytic mechanisms. Visual evidence confirming the phenomenon was later found by Noji, H. et al. (1997).

Several intracellular feedback loops, involving mitochondrial synthesis of ATP from glucose, control ATP production. Demand dictates increases or decreases in intracellular ATP levels. Cerebral neuronal synthesis and ATP usage increase during daytime activity, while neuronal production decreases during some sleep phases. The daily production and usage of googol numbers of ATP molecules makes cerebral activity possible, with small percentage changes in demand being made throughout the day and night.

Dunn, J. Grider. M.H. (2023), provide an excellent review of the topic. In what follows, I have relied on their work for much pertinent information.

The brain consumes more ATP than any other organ. One hundred to 150 moles of ATP (51 to 76Kgs) are required for normal daily human functioning, 20% of which is needed for cerebral function. The hydrolysis of ATP provides energy for a broad range of cell functions, thirty-two molecules of which are derived from the oxidation of one glucose molecule. ATP fuels the brain's synaptic signalling, cellular ion transport, chemical synthesis, impulse propagation, and DNA/RNA synthesis.

ATP is a nucleoside triphosphate, comprising a nitrogenous base (adenine), a ribose sugar, and three serially bonded phosphate groups. Deoxidation results in deoxy-ribosenucleic acid. ATP has been referred to as cellular "energy currency", energy being released with the breaking of the bond between the second and third phosphate groups. ATP synthesis utilises energy obtained from cellular respiration within the mitochondria, although beta-oxidation and ketosis are also involved. Beta-oxidation shortens fatty acid chains, yielding acetyl-CoA molecules. The catabolism of ketone bodies can also yield ATP. Catabolising glucose yields acetyl-CoA, the oxidative phosphorylation of which yields ATP.

Metabolic processes hydrolyse ATP into ADP, AMP, and free inorganic phosphate groups. ATP undergoes constant replenishment, with many feedback mechanisms maintaining consistent cellular levels. The enhancement or inhibition of ATP synthase is one regulatory mechanism. ATP inhibits phosphofructokinase-1 (PFK1) and pyruvate kinase. These two key enzymes in glycolysis act as a negative feedback loop, inhibiting glucose breakdown whenever sufficient cellular ATP is present. Because life depends so much on continuous ATP production, rather than any storage, effective feedback processes are essential.

ADP and AMP can activate PFK1 and pyruvate kinase, and promote ATP synthesis in times of high-energy demand. In the heart, ten-second bursts of activity called mitochondrial flashes, disrupt ATP production. During these demand-matched flashes, mitochondria pause ATP synthesis and release reactive oxygen species.

ATP functions as a neurotransmitter, being co-stored with acetylcholine. It also triggers the release of some hormones, various-enzymes, lipid mediators, nitric oxide, growth factors, and reactive oxygen species.

Maintaining ion concentrations across cell membranes for proper neuronal signalling, and synaptic transmission, consume ATP. Synaptic transmission is an energy-demanding process. At the presynaptic terminal, ATP is required to move neurotransmitters into vesicles and for their subsequent release. Then, ATP restores the intracellular/extracellular ion gradient in axons after each action potential. Active transport (using Na/K, ATPase) is necessary to reset the sodium, potassium, and calcium ion concentrations across cell membranes. One molecule of ATP being hydrolysed allows for three sodium ions to be transported out of the cell, and two potassium ions to be transported back into the cell, both against the concentration gradient.

One billion sodium ions (approximately) are necessary to propagate a single action potential, and nearly one billion ATP molecules need to be hydrolysed to restore the ion gradient concentration following cell depolarisation (Atwell, D. et al. 2001).

In clinical practice, intravenous ATP can act on the A1 adenosine receptor, aiding pain relief and halting some tachycardias. Adenosine compounds can reduce neuropathic pain, ischemic pain, and hyperalgesia to a level comparable to morphine. Adenosine can also decrease postoperative opioid usage, suggesting long-lasting receptor activation.

Clinicians can use ATP as a pulmonary vasodilator in patients with pulmonary hypertension and to induce hypotension during surgery. Its vasodilating effect is useful in cardiac stress imaging. It can stop triggered ventricular arrhythmias, focal atrial tachycardias, atrioventricular re-entrant tachycardia, and atrioventricular nodal re-entrant tachycardia. The European Society of Cardiology Guidelines now advocates vagal manoeuvres and adenosine as first-line interventions for supraventricular tachycardias.

The neurobiological factors described suggest a hypothesis:

- That the molecular energy available to the brain 'E', is derived from the difference between the rate of ATP energy synthesis 'S', and the contemporaneous rate of energy usage 'U', over unit time 't', modified by plasticity 'p' (see later). This ignores the very limited storage of ATP that exists (one gram total), glycogen storage with a 3-5 day turnover (glycogenolysis provides energy for ATP synthesis)(Öz. G., et al. 2007), and other forms of energy not available for immediate use.

- The dynamic molecular energy available to the healthy brain 'E' is represented by:

$$dE/dt = dS/dt - p(dU/dt)$$

Without the uncompromised drive for respiration and the control over heart rate and blood pressure, life would be unsustainable. For advanced life forms to have evolved, the synthesis of basal ganglia ATP to drive autonomic nervous system activity was essential.

Given that:

- ATP generation can respond to demand.

- ATP synthesis is unlimited.

- And the normal supply of substrate (glucose and acetyl-CoA) is unlimited,

one might speculate that the variable rate of ATP utilisation is more likely to cause TFE symptoms than its synthesis and storage.

One clinical observation supports this conclusion. The immediate restoration of perceived energy with the relief of stress is a common observation. When a major stress disappears: the winning of a court case; the moment one learns that a kidnapped victim is alive and well, there can be a rapid recovery of daytime energy and restored restorative sleep. This suggests that constant over-utilisation of neuronal energy may cause TFE symptoms that can be swiftly reversed.

Pathological conditions, such as arterial stenosis, could limit blood flow (in the absence of a collateral circulation), and could limit the delivery of glucose and oxygen to neuronal tissues, and perhaps reduce the removal of CO2. This suggests the possibility of TFE symptoms arising from cerebral atherosclerosis and ischaemia. This has been shown to be the case (Jolly. A.A. et al. 2024). The atheroma present would have to be ubiquitous and obstructive in cerebral arteries, given the several alternative sources of blood supply available from the Circle of Willis.

Extreme tiredness ('vital exhaustion') is a known feature of established dementia, and is useful as a premonitory sign (Islamoska, S., et al. 2019). In such cases, neuronal malfunctioning is likely to involve disturbed synaptic function and axonal transmission, with disturbed ATP synthesis (Zhang, C. et al. 2015).

Interruption of neuronal activity also occurs with inflammatory plaque formation in multiple sclerosis (MS). This involves myelin destruction and axonal degeneration in the brain and spinal cord..

Tiredness is the commonest symptom (Braley, T.J. & Chervin, R. D. 2010). As in chronic fatigue syndrome, it can be associated with decreased cortisol (Cleare, A.J. 2003) and DHEA levels (Maes, M. et al. 2005).

Chapter Three

Neurotransmitters and TFE Symptoms

The discovery of the action potential and synaptic transmission at the neuromuscular junction by Emil du Bois-Reymond (1848–1884), was a landmark moment in neurophysiology (Finkelstein, G. 2015). His discovery led to our current understanding of how electrical energy activates the heart and brain. By 1969, researchers had discovered that calcium triggered presynaptic transmitter vesicle discharge, leading to synaptic transmission and depolarisation of the post-synapse.

An action potential arriving at a presynaptic terminal releases transmitters from vesicles in under one millisecond. This is enabled by Ca2+ influx binding to synaptotagmin (a family of N-terminal and cytoplasmic proteins). Linked to SNARE and SN proteins, vesicles fuse with the synaptic membrane (Südhof, T.C. 2013).

In the brain, several transmitters are available. Which they are, depends on the area of the brain and its global cerebral function – sleep, wakefulness, cognition, emotion, memory, decision making, and action. They include acetylcholine (the first transmitter to be discovered), nor-epinephrine, serotonin, glutamate, ATP, GABA, and dopamine.

Understanding how TFE symptoms arise and how they might be treated, requires more than the understanding of neurotransmitter function. The global functioning of the brain results from the integration of many neurophysiological processes. Using the word 'complex' as defined by Hayek (Hayek, F.A. 1967), the processes that enable physiological homeostasis, consciousness, emotional reactions, logical deduction, and decision making are complex. This results from the involvement of many interconnected variables, acting both dependently and independently, at any one time.

What follows is a brief review of transmitters and how they function, with special attention to stress, sleep, and wakefulness.

Acetylcholine (ACh)

Acetylcholine is a ubiquitous transmitter, found in neuromuscular junctions, in the autonomic system, the basal forebrain, and brainstem (mesopontine tegmentum) areas. Two ACh receptor types exist, each with subtypes: nicotinic (ionotropic, depolarising) and muscarinic (metabolic). The role of ACh in the brain is not fully understood, but is involved in memory, arousal, and attention.

Although ACh is active at neuromuscular junctions and in autonomic ganglia, in the brain it acts as a neuromodulator, affecting synaptic plasticity. It can increase neurotransmitter release, promoting burst firing and suppressing tonic firing (Piciotto, M.R. et al. 2012).

In mammals, cholinergic mechanisms are not alone in controlling sleep. Monoamines, glutamate, GABA, serotonine, and dopamine all have a part to play in different regions of the brain, sometimes inter-reacting with melatonin. Dopamine, for instance, with its receptors and neurones, promotes wakefulness and arousal to stimuli. ACh receptor agonists like nicotine can enhance the cognitive processes of animals (Pirikh, V., et al 2008), and enhance cognition in patients (Wilens, T.E. et al. 2007).

The brain contains various cholinergic receptors (13 in Drosophila). Some are responsible for arousal, and others for sleep. (Dai, X. et al. 2021). In humans, the role played by ACh receptors in arousal and sleep is largely unknown. Specific parts of the brain are involved. For instance, in the locus coeruleus, ACh receptors modify norepinephrine release as part of the ascending arousal system. These are most active during REM sleep and wakefulness.

Recent genetic studies in mice have revealed ACh receptor phenotypes which predispose to sleep and wakefulness. Mutation studies reveal how various receptor phenotypes can lead to a complete loss of REM sleep, decreased sleep duration, and reduced non-REM sleep (Niwa, Y. et al. 2018).

The depolarisation of neurones and the resulting waveforms, conducted throughout the brain, are sometimes ACh dependent. Na+ and Ca2+ influx activates the post-synaptic junction, making some electrical brain activity ACh dependent. The phasic release of ACh over seconds, can define cognitive operations (Sartar, M. et al. 2009), but it will also work in concert with other neuro-transmitters like ATP, serotonin, nor-epinephrine, dopamine (Briand, L.A. et al. 2007) and the inhibitory transmitter GABA (gamma-aminobutyric acid)(Saunders, A. et al. 2015). In the rat cerebral cortex, the density of cholinergic activity is similar throughout (Lysakowski, A. et al. 1989).

Two models of ACh activity exist:

- The 'wired model', accepts the rapid release, activation, and hydrolysis of ACh by acetyl-cholinesterase (ACHE).

- In the volume model, free ACh is available to activate other cells (equivalent to electronic induction perhaps).

Both occur, but in different parts of the brain.

In the pre-synaptic terminal, choline acetyltransferase (CHAT) catalyses the synthesis of ACh from choline and acetyl CoA. Acetylcholine transporter (VACHT) then packs ACh into vesicles, released on depolarisation of the terminal. Following release, ACh can bind to receptors (nicotinic and muscarinic) where it is rapidly hydrolysed by acetyl-cholinesterase (ACHE), to yield choline and acetate. Most cortical ACh remains free to activate other neurones.

When ACHE is inactivated, ACh levels can rise one hundred-fold (Sartar, M. et al. 2009). ACHE clustering at the synapse allows hydrolysis of 5000 molecules of ACh per second. Its activity and presence in different parts of the brain are not fully known. Its rapid hydrolysing capability suggests that the volume theory of transmission is relevant only in its absence.

In heart pacemaker cells, depolarisation results from the repeated slow influx of K+. The change of conductance is modified by autonomic ACh and nor-epinephrine. Theoretically, sinus bradycardia and AV block could result from defective ACHE (as in diphtheria). This has been seen to occur in rabbits with diphtheritic myocarditis ((Malivanova, S.D. 1968). Diphtheria toxin is an anticholinesterase)(Dighton. D.H. 1974).

Because the heart never stops throughout life, and can sustain a heart rate of 120bpm (one beat every half-second), pre-synaptic ACh must be constantly and reliably replenished. Like ATP production, its synthesis is likely to be conserved and almost infinite in relation to requirements. Life would not be possible otherwise. In fact, the replenishing time for pre-synaptic ACh (and NE) needs at least to be 0.5secs (with a heart rate of 120bpm). If the same priorities hold true for brain ACh replenishment, it would seem unlikely that ACh depletion is a cause for TFE symptoms in normal patients. Because anti-cholinesterase drugs (donepezil, rivastigmine, and galantamine) improve cognitive function in dementia (Singh, R. 2023), TFE in cerebral ischaemia and amyloid must relate to ACh depletion. Its inactivation, or abnormal ACHE activity are also possible.

Reduced cerebrospinal levels of acetylcholine (ACh) are found in those with Alzheimer's disease (AD). The concentration correlated with the degree of dementia (Toghi, H., et al. 1994).

In the axon terminal pre-synapse, newly formed acetylcholine is collected in vesicles, with very few molecules remaining free in the axon cytosol. The vesicles are acidified via an energy-dependent H-ATPase pump. This creates a gradient for acetylcholine to enter vesicles using vesicular acetylcholine transporter (VAChT). One vesicular proton (H+) is exchanged for each molecule of acetylcholine (Muramatsu, I. et al. 2018).

Ach Synthesis

In the foetus, ACh is found in the first moments of the developing ectoderm (neural plate), its actions being fundamental to neural cell differentiation.

For the synthesis of acetylcholine, CAT catalyses the reaction of choline with acetyl-CoA. CAT is produced in the neuronal soma (body) and transported to synapses by axoplasmic transport. Vesicles full of various proteins are attach to actin filaments that span the length of the neuron. Although localised to the axon terminus, CAT is present throughout the neuron (Leuzinger, W. 1969).

Alzheimer dementia patients, but not those with ischaemic dementia, can have a reduced cerebral content of choline acetyltransferase (CAT)(Wilcock, G.K. et al.(1982), decreased acetylcholine synthesis, and impaired cortical cholinergic function. The severity of dementia relates to the decrease of CAT activity, but could a reduction in ACh synthesis account for TFE symptoms?

Nor-epinephrine (NE)

Nor-epinephrine (NE) is a mono-amine synthesised from dopamine. Found mainly in the pons and medulla, the locus ceoruleous is a main area for its production. NE is the main transmitter of sympathetic ganglia in the spinal cord, but is also released from the adrenal medulla. It acts on G-protein coupled adrenergic receptors (alpha-1, alpha-2 and beta-receptors), each of which have several sub-types. It is removed from the synaptic cleft by NE transporter. Like ACh, NE is also associated with memory, arousal, attention, and the complex physiological effects associated with stress; in particular, fight and flight.

NE is most likely to be involved in the cognitive drive to solve those long-term, stressful problems, typical of many TFE patients.

Serotonin

Serotonin is a monoamine neurotransmitter derived from L-tryptophan. It is converted to 5-hydroxy-tryptophan (5-HTP) and then to 5-hydroxytryptomine (5-HT) or serotonin. Serotonin producing neurones are found mainly in the brainstem's raphe nuclei. From there, they influence many parts of the brain. There are seven families of serotonin receptors (5HT-1R to 5HT-7R).

They have some of the following features:

- 5HT-1R and 5R receptors are inhibitory. They inhibit cAMP production and cause K+ efflux, making depolarisation less likely. They also close Ca2+ channels.
- 5HT-4, 6 & 7R are excitatory. They may increase cAMP levels and close K+ channels.
- 5HT-2R allows Ca2+ influx.
- 5HT-3R is ionotropic. It allows Na+ influx and makes depolarisation more likely.

A re-uptake transporter protein (SERT removes serotonin from the synaptic cleft). Deficient serotonin causes depression; therefore, when antidepressants increase SERT persistence and thus serotonin levels, mood improves and depression lessens. These effects are exaggerated when patients also take St. John's Wort.

Serotonin can diffuse outside of the synaptic cleft to influence other areas. This effect can make other synapses more liable to depolarise.

Stimulating the HT-1R receptor can have antipsychotic, anti-depressant and anti-anxiety effects. Blocking the HT-1R receptor can also act as an antidepressant. The effect depends on whether it is acting in the pre- or post-synapse, and where in the brain. This makes the clinical functioning of serotonin receptors complex.

Over the last twenty years, the understanding of 5HT receptors has progressed. For animal and human brains, atlases of 5-HT receptor distribution are available. 5-HT receptors reside within complex neural circuits. Unexpected complexity in 5-HT receptor function has been identified, including agonist-dependent signalling. Combined 5-HT signalling and co-released neurotransmitters (especially glutamate) also occur.

Much more needs to be known about how 5-HT receptor types interact with complex neural circuits, to generate the neurophysiological changes that lead to altered cognition and behaviour (Sharp, T., Barnes, N.M. 2020).

The mood changes associated with TFE symptoms are likely to involve changes in serotonin and 5-HT receptors. It is not surprising, therefore, that symptoms of depression and those occurring during TFE (in those not subject to depression), have similarities.

Dopamine

Dopamine is a catecholamine formed from the amino acid tyrosine being converted to L-DOPA, and then carboxylated to dopamine. It is found in the substantia nigra, ventral tegmental area, hypothalamus, retina, and olfactory bulb. The nigrostriatal, mesolimbic and meso-cortical tuberoinfundibular pathways carry dopamine to the cortex. At least five dopamine receptors populate the system. A specific transporter removes dopamine from the synaptic cleft.

Dopamine is associated with movement, learning motor skills, rewarding and pleasurable experiences, and the coordination required for executive functioning. It is also involved in arousal, sleep, attention, motivation, and adaptive behaviour. It is, therefore, likely to be involved in the generation of TFE symptoms.

GABA

Gamma-amino-butyric acid is an inhibitory neurotransmitter. It binds to post-synaptic regions. By modulating ion transport, it causes hyperpolarisation and thus inhibits depolarisation.

It is synthesised in the pre-synapse from glutamate, with pyridoxine (vitamin B6) as a co-factor. Like other transmitters, it is stored in pre-synaptic vesicles. Once released, it can either bind to post-synaptic receptors, be degraded by GABA transaminase, or be reabsorbed back into the pre-synapse.

There are two major receptors:

- GABA-A allows the uptake of (negative) Cl- ions which hyperpolarise the cell and inhibit depolarisation.

- GABA-B receptors cause inhibitory hyperpolarisation. They increase the conductance of K+ and decrease the conductance of Ca2+ ions.

For treating some neurological and psychiatric conditions, modulation of GABA signalling has been found effective. In the medulla, GABA governs respiratory rate. With increasing GABA, respiratory rate reduces. Huntingdon's Chorea, hepatic encephalopathy, dystonia, and spasticity, can all include a GABA related component. Diazepam, by involving the GABA-A receptor, increases Cl- ion permeability. Perhaps because alcohol affects same receptors, diazepam has been found useful in alcohol withdrawal.

Because sleep enforced with diazepam helps to reverse the more severe cases of TFE (from my personal experience), it is possible that GABA receptors are involved in the aetiology of TFE symptoms.

Glutamate

Glutamate is an important neurotransmitter, found mostly in the hippocampus and cerebral cortex. Like other transmitters, it is stored in pre-synaptic vesicles. In his book: The Organisation of Behaviour. A Neuropsychological Theory. (Routledge. 1949), Donald O. Hebb correctly postulated that if connected neurones fire together in a coordinated manner, their connection strengthens; when uncoordinated, their connections weaken.

It is now known that the strengthening and weakening of transmission (plasticity), depends on which fires first – the pre- or post-synapse (https://qbi.uq.edu.au/brain-basics/brain/brain-physiology/long-term-synaptic-plasticity, provides a summary). If the presynaptic dendrite fires first (20msecs before the post-synaptic), transmission strengthens (so called long-term potentiation); the reverse occurs when the post-synaptic dendrite fires first: it causes long-term depression.

The post-synaptic receptors are either metabolic or ion-channel. The latter can open or close, be excitatory (glutamate related), or inhibitory. Two glutamate receptors are known:

- AMPA (alpha-amino-3 hydroxy-5 methyl-4 isoxazolepropionic acid) that depolarises cells through Na+ and K+ flux, and,

- NMDA (N-methyl-d aspartate) that magnesium ions can block.

In the hippocampus, it is glutamate that depolarises the post-synaptic dendrites via AMPA receptors. After the cell depolarises, NMDA receptors become activated, allowing an influx of Ca2+ ions.

Depolarisation of the cell activates both receptor types, causing Na+, K+ and Ca2+ ions to flow. Ca2+ ion flow determines plasticity (the up- and down-scaling of synaptic transmission). A large

Ca2+ influx leads to potentiation; a decreased Ca2+ influx leads to long-term suppression. If the post-synaptic dendrite fires first, Ca2+ ion flux occurs in fewer NMDA receptors.

Ca2+ ions in large numbers activate kinases and increase the number of AMPA receptors. Phosphatases, activated by lower Ca2+ fluxes, result in fewer AMPA receptors being recycled. AMPA receptors are recycled from the synaptic cleft. They travel around, then backwards into the axon cell.

The up- and down-scaling of transmission (synaptic strength), is called homeostatic plasticity, a basic neural network function, related to adaptive behaviour (Turrigiano, G.G. 2004). Sleep modulates synaptic plasticity. Diekelmann, S. (2010) and Kuhn. M., et al (2016), showed that sleep recalibrates synaptic plasticity. In the human brain, sleep deprivation reduces plasticity by increasing synaptic strength (increased current and voltage in the post-synaptic neurones). This is associated with an increase in ACh vesicle numbers, and more ACh released into the synaptic cleft. This process is likely involved in the natural history of TFE symptoms.

Sleep is thought to occur when the whole brain exhibits slow-wave activity. In the sleep-deprived subjects, however, only small areas of the brain exhibit slow wave outputs—a few areas of the brain that are partially asleep. One area that does this is the thalamic reticular nucleus (TRN) that surrounds the thalamus. When active enough, it can control the entire brain (as in coma and anaesthesia)(Voigts, J., et al. 2015).

Sleep is associated with the down-scaling of synaptic strength. Once synapses have been saturated by wakefulness, sleep recalibrates them. Certain experiences will saturate synapses so that no further learning can occur from their involvement (Nguyen-Vu, T.D.B. 2017). Sleep-associated down-scaling may improve signal-noise ratio and improve the capacity to encode new information (Tononi, G. 2014). The defective sleep associated with TFE symptoms could interfere with this process.

TFE patients often have defective sleep and impaired cognitive function. Could a reduction in synaptic down-scaling explain this?

In mice, the plasticity of neurones (in specific muscarinic receptor sub-types), relates to ACh concentration and cholinesterase activity (Kuczewski, N. 2005). Long-term, glutamatergic transmission is liable to saturation, with feedback that can decrease it. Could greater degrees of tiredness (from tiredness to exhaustion) be related to these processes, increasing within the stressed, sleep-deprived brain (hypothalamus)?

Although we cannot yet measure such processes in humans, some indirect observations may prove relevant. The EEG response to magnetic stimulation increases with time awake and is reset by sleep (Huber, R. et al. 2012). EEG theta activity (and the need for sleep) increases with time awake. The significance of such observations to the neuronal activities described remains the subject of further research.

Melatonin

The pineal gland receives information about ambient light conditions and produces melatonin in response. The pineal gland may not be 'the seat of the soul', as suggested by René Descartes, but it does direct circadian physiology. Importantly, for the understanding of TFE symptoms, it can control the timing of wakefulness and the need for sleep. Therapeutically, it has been used for delayed sleep-phase syndrome, non-2-hour sleep-wake disorder, and jet-lag. During the day, blood levels of melatonin are usually undetectable.

The pineal gland produces melatonin under dark external conditions (sensed by retinal connections). Tryptophan is converted to 5-hydroxytryptophan (5-HTP); 5-HTP is converted to 5-HT, and thereafter converted to N-acetyl serotonin, then melatonin (Gastel, J.A. et al. 1998). When light reaches the pineal gland, melatonin production stops. The process depends on light reaching the pineal via the suprachiasmatic nucleus (SCN). The SCN then secretes GABA. GABA then inhibits the paraventricular nucleus (PVN) of the hypothalamus, which inhibits pineal melatonin production.

Arendt and Aulinas have pointed to a new mechanism (Arendt, J. Aulinas, A. 2022). In mouse brains, melatonin is only synthesised in mitochondria. In the cytoplasm, this can activate a mitochondrial MT1 signal-transduction pathway, inhibiting stress-mediated cytochrome-c release and caspase activation. As a prelude to cell death and inflammation, melatonin might thus protect against neurodegeneration (Suofu, Y. et al. 2017).

Jet-lag and insomnia disturb melatonin production. Its dysfunction is therefore likely to be involved in the aetiology and maintenance of TFE symptoms. This raises the question of its use in those with TFE symptoms.

I well remember both a lorry driver and a young woman, both complaining of undue tiredness during the day. At night they were both active and alert. Their circadian rhythm was out of phase with the majority, most of whom are active in the morning. The lorry driver solved his problem by driving only at night. The young woman solved hers by becoming a croupier and working the early shift between midnight and daybreak.

When I explained sleep being out of phase to an entrepreneur business executive, he was quick to see an advantage over others. He asked, 'Does that mean that if I hold important business meetings late on Friday afternoon, I will gain the mental advantage over others?'

Chapter Four

Bio-Physical Neurophysiology

The current outlook, made popular by newsfeeds and social media, is that computers and AI are more valuable, and hold more promise to help humanity, than brains. Computers can calculate, search data, organise and decide on a probability basis faster than any human brain. Human brains, however, can create anew (not just by sampling known ideas). We can use thinking, emotion and personal experience to make wise judgements that can benefit individuals, not just the average person, represented by a large group.

Alan Türing, who invented the test to judge whether a computer could be accepted as human, declared the question "too meaningless" for discussion. He thought the best computers could only play an imitation game (Türing, A. 1950). The philosopher J. Searle, by proposing the Chinese room experiment, demonstrates that a computer program does not need to understand or think in order to be thought capable of understanding and thinking.

We do not need to compare apples to pears, or brains to computers. They both bring separate value. To understand relative value, we need to understand how both function. Before considering their physical functioning, consider some general points.

Our brains are ionic organs activated by cations, with one extra proton (Na+ and K+), or two (Mg2+; Ca2+), with Cl as an anion, playing a minor role. Computers are electron-driven devices that can function at light speed; brain function is restricted by action potential transmission (approximately 52 – 80 metres/sec)(Macefield, G. et al. 1989).

In what became the most admired products of the human brain, speed never featured. It took Einstein half of his lifetime to formulate his theory of relativity, and Tesla's conception of AC current took rather longer than a day! Michelangelo's creations suffered nothing from the time he took to create them (although his sponsors might have disagreed). Contrast this with the speed of computer processing, that allows almost instantaneous calculation, essential for navigation using GPS, or for Forex trading. Like apples and pears, brains, and computers need only be complimentary. Obviously, no matter how much a pear aspires to be an apple, or vice versa, it can only happen as an illusion.

Although one brain resembles all others, and computers share much of the same architecture, computers and brains have little in common other than some functional connectivity. Brains require the complex functioning of diversely connected neuronal networks to allow thinking, emotion, and wise decision-making. Uniqueness lies within the variability of neuronal connection. Computers are all made to a blueprint. Computers are complicated, but they use fixed wired circuits, able only to process data according to instructions (programs) that human brains design.

Brains need rest, computers do not (as long as their cooling devices and power supply remain functioning. Airports and hospitals, however, are occasionally brought to a dangerous halt because their computers cannot function without power. Their physical components can fail, and their systems are soon obsolete without human intervention. Can any computer be made reliable enough to take charge of a life?

The brain, as an organised physical system, somewhat parallels electronic circuitry. Brains came first, and from their educated functioning, electronic circuits were born and developed. Some believe the reverse to be possible: computers designing themselves. Both brains and all physical systems (including computers) must obey the same principles, as first pointed out by Emil du Bois-Reymond (1848–1884)(Finkelstein, G. 2015), but there the analogy ends.

In electronic circuits, wires, switches, resistors, capacitors, inductors, and energy generators, all have a physical form. No equivalent of a battery as a single organ exists in the brain. Instead, each cell acts as a battery with energy delivered through chemical processes using high-energy ATP molecules. Synapses exist rather than switches or diodes; transmitters are transported against the resistance of dendritic spines, rather than having circuit resistors; stored transmitter vesicles, rather than capacitors; some synaptic transmitters escaping to affect other cells, rather than fixed, hard-wired inductors.

In electronic circuits, electrons provide the current. In axons, it is proton influx (Na+ ions) that initiates every action potential, and can travel many paths through a network of neurones in the brain. Electronic circuits can also collect or emit light, deliver chemicals, or measure light, heat, and pH. Unlike electronic circuits, the brain releases neurotransmitters like ACh, serotonin, and dopamine, to influence consciousness, mood, and attention.

Could hardware circuitry ever achieve consciousness? Computer hardware may seem complicated, but complex brain configuration and neuronal interconnectivity remain unmatched. Equally unmatched, are their functioning and outputs. Since human and animal consciousness arises from an unrivalled complex system, no electronic device so far devised, is likely to achieve it. No need exists. The brain and electro-mechanical systems are equivalent, but constructed differently. Any consciousness achieved by a machine would have separate features; ones that incorporate fast processing (sorting, matching, and calculation), but ring-fenced by their engineered design, their need for algorithmic control, and in the future, decision pathways dictated only by probability calculations (AI). Any such 'consciousness' would be quite unlike the human sort, but could be complementary. TFE symptoms can modify consciousness: something, machines need not experience.

In all physical systems, scale is an important consideration. Rules applicable to one scale may not apply to another. The behaviour of sub-atomic particles, for instance, does not predict the movement of bodies in the Newtonian world of physics (and vice versa). The cellular actions of ions and molecules in axons and synapses is one thing, but the integrated actions and interactions of neurones function at a global scale. Global cerebral functioning enables perceiving, thinking, feeling, and reacting to events. This functioning is far removed in scale from the movement of transmitters across synaptic gaps. Machines also function at different scales, but are less complicated, and programmed with instructions that introduce self-limitation and obsolescence. Software limits govern global computer function, regardless of outward appearances, making it predictable (at least to programmers). While they may draw attention to surprising combinations, and produce unforeseen output, one must not misinterpret these as acts of de novo creation.

Non-REM sleep is associated with slow-wave (low power) activity. Less power dissipation implies less synaptic activity or more inhibition. Wakefulness is associated with more power dissipation, recorded as EEG waves of greater amplitude and frequency, most likely generated by an increase in synaptic activity or its potentiation. A key characteristic of many synapses is use dependence.

'One of the most important and fascinating properties of the mammalian brain is its plasticity; the capacity of the neural activity generated by an experience, to modify neural circuit function and thereby modify subsequent thoughts, feelings, and behaviour.' (Citri, A. & Malenka, R.C. 2007).

From the start, AI development has attempted to follow in the footsteps of neuronal functioning.

Switches and Synapses

Synapses are not simple switches, like those found in electronic circuits; they have 'plasticity' and strength and are variable. They can reduce transmission through reduced receptor or synapse numbers (age and dementia; receptor recycling), and by the downregulation of the synapses that remain (Berchtold, N. et al. 2012). Hyper-polarisation, post-synaptic feedback action potentials, and inhibitory neurones can all reduce transmission. Berchtold, et al. also noted changes in: 'synaptic vesicle trafficking and release, neurotransmitter receptors, receptor trafficking, postsynaptic density scaffolding, cell adhesion regulating synaptic stability, and neuro-modulatory systems.' Presynaptic vesicles can get depleted, with receptor numbers subject to change. Desensitisation of ligand-gated receptors, making the target neuron less sensitive to neurotransmitter, also occurs (Citri, A., & Malenka, R.C. 2008). In addition, inhibitory synapses undergo constant turnover (Villa. K.L. et al. 2016).

Ca2+ ion flow determines plasticity (the up- and down-scaling of synaptic transmission). A large Ca2+ influx leads to potentiation; decreased Ca2+ influx leads to long-term depression. If the post-synaptic dendrite fires first, Ca2+ ion flux takes place in fewer NMDA receptors.

The dendritic spines on which synapses sit, can amplify signals through changes in conductance (Harnett, M.T. et al. 2013), but potentiation (Hao, J. et al. 2012), and the increased frequency of transmission also occur (Turrigiano, G.G. 2004). With use, some synapses adapt and become inhibited. Does wakefulness diminish the number of transmitting synapses, later to be re-set during sleep?

Since no limit exists for the amount of ATP energy available to cells, the concepts of a 'flat battery' or 'burn-out' have no neurophysiological basis. Restriction of high-energy ATP availability could cause TFE symptoms, except no evidence exists for the limited synthesis of either ATP or neurotransmitters. Because the cessation of respiration and heart pacemaker function would be incompatible with life, only death will switch off the supply of molecular energy required for synaptic transmission in the brain stem. From the evolutionary perspective, less vital cerebral functions, like cognition and emotion, might be different, perhaps switching energy supply on and off as required.

If we consider fully sentient human functioning, there are physical principles useful as metaphors for understanding behaviour and clinical outcomes. In the same way that elastic is lengthened (a strain effect) by attaching a weight (a stressor), humans who experience stress can also respond. Humans can react to the same stress in different ways, depending on their constitution, learning and experience (weak or strong elastic provides a useful analogy). Stretched enough, all elastic snaps, regardless of its constitution. Some situations are cliff edge, bi-stable phenomena; the equivalent to elastic snapping. When standing close to a high cliff edge, one need only take one small step to end up in pieces. The sudden occurrence of heart attacks, strokes, immune problems leading to infection, psychosis, and mental illnesses can all represent catastrophic medical phenomena.

In a physics laboratory, defined entities like energy, power, stress, and strain are measurable. Analogy alone makes it possible to apply simple mechanical principles to biological systems. Human beings can undergo cognitive, emotional, and physical stress. Although the stressors and the biological responses can be generalised, our responses are usually individual. In biological terms, one could refer to elastic strength as 'constitution': a characteristic encompassing physical and mental strength, adaptability, and a capacity for functional efficiency.

Clinicians might accept the stress-strain relationship in principle, but patients may view applied forces differently, and have different reactions. Bereavement, bankruptcy, or divorce will affect some more than others. Although all such non-standard incidents (applied forces) have either to be coped with or ignored, the amount of emotion or cognitive concern they raise (strain effects), will differ between individuals. Stressful situations can affect different physiological systems, like sleep, immunity, heart rate control, blood pressure, and blood coagulability. The 'strain' effects may vary with genetic predisposition. In this way, a stressed hypertensive patient can become resistant to treatment. Blood pressure might become uncontrollable during an acrimonious divorce or through bankruptcy. Many others will have no change in their blood pressure whatsoever.

Unlike a weight tied to a piece of elastic, biological systems are not simple. Instead, they are dynamic, requiring energy to be spent on maintaining homeostasis. In the brain, different reactions may be involved, most of which include the release of energy from the breakdown of ATP. Different areas of the brain will release varying amounts of energy and utilise it in different ways, causing distinct waves of depolarisation to be integrated and recorded as EEGs (with varying frequency and amplitude).

In simple electronic circuitry, LCR circuits that create pulses are of interest. A circuit containing a resistor (R), a capacitor (C), and an induction coil (L), will produce voltage waves similar to those of an EEG (electronic ringing circuits). When the circuit current is off, or between voltage pulses, electrons reverberate between the two energy reserving components: the capacitor, and the induction coil. This produces a sinusoidal voltage/current wave. As with AC current, these waves represent different levels of power generation.

In those patients without TFE, the more aroused the person, the greater the power expressed by their EEG. In the quieter phases of NREM sleep, the frequency (f) and amplitude (A) of brain waves become attenuated. This represents reduced power usage, where power (P) = $2\pi fA$.

Since the normal supply of ATP is all but limitless, any perception of TFE symptoms must relate to energy availability and use, the effects of neurotransmitters or hormone release. At a global level, local release of serotonin, dopamine, glutamate, nor-adrenaline, acetylcholine, and melatonin can all alter mood and the perception of TFE symptoms.

Any systemic release of cortisol, oestrogen, progesterone, and endorphins will combine their effects with local ones. Cortisol levels slowly increase during the second half of the sleep period. Growth hormone peaks during the first half of sleep; prolactin peaks in the middle of the sleep period and decreases with awakening. TSH secretion increases during sleep, while the secretion of triiodothyronine (T3) and thyroxine (T4) decreases. It has been suggested that hypothalamic growth hormone-releasing hormone (GHRH) promotes sleep, while corticotropin-releasing hormone promotes awakening and wakefulness. Sleep deprivation increases insulin resistance, decreases leptin (to inhibit hunger), and increases gherlin (stimulates hunger)(Mascetti, G.G. 2016).

In chapter 2, I hypothesised that at the global level, our perceived mental energy 'E', must derive from the amount of cellular energy (ATP) being synthesised 'S', minus its usage 'U', its availability being controlled through variants of synaptic plasticity 'p'. We can represent the dynamic situation in healthy adults by:

$$dE/dt = dS/dt - p(dU/dt)$$

Since the storage of ATP is insignificant, the cellular component 'S' is a key variable, but the availability of energy at a molecular level being continuously controlled by synaptic plasticity (Turrigiano, G.G. 2004). EEG waveforms represent a function of brain power being used (dE/dt; related to amplitude and frequency). 'E' rises with daytime wakefulness and diminishes to its lowest during NREM sleep (Fig. 3). The variable 'U' – energy usage – is also a key component. I wonder if, in high demand situations, the perception of energy usage could provide feedback that might vary perceived TFE symptoms?

The mechanism of energy restoration achieved by restful sleep remains a mystery. Could it relate to the un-blocking and re-setting of synapses, since it is most unlikely to relate to either ATP production or storage? Patterns of inherent brain activity that activate optimism and ego on one hand, and depression and demoralisation on the other, can boost or reduce the perception of 'having energy'.

PART TWO

Chapter Five

Ancient and Modern Views of Sleep

The Divine Panacea?

It would seem that views about sleep have changed little in time. They range from believing that healing gods would visit in sleep to a time for organising memories and thoughts. Portrayals of sleep as healing, restful, and recharging appear in Greek mythology, the Bible, and art from the Renaissance to the modern era. Also, it is a vulnerable state, a time when reasoning is absent and dreams might reveal secrets. Refreshing, untroubled sleep, is now recognised as important for mental health. There is nothing new about the relationship between continuing unresolved stress, TFE symptoms, and an inability to sleep well. I have referred to this as the sleep paradox: when refreshing sleep is most needed, it is least likely to happen. Sleep EEGs during this time resemble those during wakefulness. It has thus been called paradoxical sleep.

What follows are snapshots of the depiction and understanding of sleep and dreaming throughout history.

Ancient Greek, pre-Socratic, and Hippocratic writers traced the ability of wine to promote or disturb sleep (Magowan, S.R. 2017). Ancient Greek writers described wine as a 'refuge from troubles' (τὸν καμάτων λιμένα). In her academic thesis, Magowan points to the under-rated significance of these writers, many of whom linked sleep to divine activity (Hypnos, Thanatos, Hermes, Asclepius); some of whom (Hippocratic writers) made a profession of dream interpretation. In what follows, I have relied on Magowan's thesis for ancient views of sleep function.

In Ancient Greece, Aristotle thought that while sleeping, one entered the borderland between life and death. It was also thought that the sick were visited by Morpheus during sleep; sleep being a divine panacea.

In Sophocles' Philoctetes: there is a hymn to sleep which highlights its pain-relief and healing quality:

'O Sleep, unknowing of pains, O Sleep, unknowing of suffering! May you come to us in favour, fortunate, Giver of happy life, lord! May you continue to hold before his eyes This light, which now has been spread over them. Come, come, Healer!'

The hymn, delivered is part of a deception (Philoctetes), was not meant to be genuine.

That sleep took on a particularly curative role in tragedy, appears in a brief fragment from Sophocles' Eriphyle. 'The old man warns that Heracles must not be woken from his sleep as it will stir and rouse up the 'dreadful sickness' that is afflicting him (δεινὴν νόσον)'.

Sleep, as a form of 'release' during times of duress, was thought elusive. Magowan makes the point that 'from Homer onwards, characters suffer from insomnia on account of their overactive psychological organs. This is an affliction which besets both immortals and mortals indiscriminately.'

Sleep deprivation and other hardships (ἀγωγά - agoga) were integral to Spartan education for all males between the ages of seven and thirty years.

In ancient Greece, Hypnos was the god of sleep, and people believed Hermes could induce sleep and wakefulness with his golden staff. The Iliad describes Hermes as capable of lulling anyone to sleep. Athena was said to ease the sufferings of Penelope and Odysseus, separated for twenty years. During Odysseus' absence, Penelope mourned, fearing her suitors, and worrying about her future. Her (disturbed) sleep did not, however, release her from stress (Homer. The Odyssey).

The combined duties of Hypnos and Thanatos reflected a close association between sleep and death. Zeus, for example, sent dreams, such as the 'destructive dream' (οὖλον ὄνειρον) he sent Agamemnon, convincing him to launch a fateful attack on the Trojans without Achilles. Some early writers thought dreams to exist as multiple entities: a tribe, a race of their own, with a shared identity.

A common epithet was applied by early Greek writers to sleep: that it was 'sweet' (γλύκυς - glykis, from which 'glucose' is derived). Zeus' own sleep was described as γλύκυς; Agamemnon's sleep as ἀμβρόσιος ('ambrosial'). Others described sleep as cruel (σχέτλιος, or 'terrible' (δεινὸν).

Sophocles suggests that sleep wields temporary power over even the highest of immortals, as a state of vulnerability. Euripides' Hecuba, describes Trojans overcome by 'sweet sleep' after dinner (ὕπνος ἡδὺς), unaware of the disaster about to befall them. In contrast to the noise and anxiety of war, peace offers the possibility of undisturbed sleep. People thought that a 'forgetful' state of sleep induced by the gods would provide a temporary respite from suffering. They recognised how stress affects sleep, and how sleep helps to cope with stress.

Clytemnestra, Agamemnon's wife, the ancient world's most wronged woman, attempts to rouse the Furies from their slumber. She warns them not to be 'softened' by sleep or lulled into an ignorance of miseries (μηδ' ἀγνοήσῃς πῆμα μαλθαχθεῖσ' ὕπνῳ).

On many occasions, fear is mentioned as a root cause of insomnia. Those kept awake are most often fearful of future suffering.

In cases of extreme emotional or psychological turbulence, sleep is seen as elusive without the intervention of gods. The sleeping state has the inherent potential to release us from stress and harm (disquiet), during ongoing suffering. In the Odyssey, Homer makes clear that for Penelope, 'sleep brings a pause to lamenting, and a forgetfulness of all things, good and bad'. The sleeper, however, is vulnerable to dreaming.

Magowan points out that analysing and categorising ancient views of dreams is problematic. 'It is culturally manipulative to try and force universal categories upon dreams from ancient to modern societies; there are, of course, similarities in content but this can be culturally subjective, i.e. that which symbolises good fortune in one culture may mean the complete opposite in another.' A fearful dream for one person, may not be troublesome to another.

Ancient Greeks commonly distinguished between internal and external dreams, the former being symbolic or episodic, the latter featuring direct interactions with a visiting figure.

'A man in the night kindles a light for himself, his eyes having been extinguished; living, he touches that which is dead while sleeping; having woken, he touches that which is sleeping.'

In this fragment, the link between the two conscious states suggests that the kindled light (created in sleep), shows the preservation of life within man, and differentiates life from death.

Heraclitus plays with this notion:

θάνατός ἐστιν ὁκόσα ἐγερθέντες ὁρέομεν, ὁκόσα δὲ εὕδοντες ὕπνος.
Death is all we see when awake, while all we see when sleeping is sleep.

Insomnia once referred to the sharing of political equality and was an ancient term for Athenian demokratia. Alcmaeon used it to recognise primary political sense; 'the nearest comparative use in Herodotus, places it in direct comparison to both tyranny and democracy.' The thinking was the 'equilibrium of oppositional powers, is what sustains health.' (Magowan, S.R. 2017).

Alcmaeon believed that the movement of blood brought about sleep. Anaxagoras says, sleep happens because of weariness from bodily activity; an experience of the body, not of the soul. Sleep is seen as a 'practice run' for death – the term διδασκαλίας – related to teaching, lessons, and rehearsals in a theatre.

As an example of ancient physiological misconception, Diogenes believed that as blood fills the veins, the air in them is pushed into the chest and belly beneath it. He thought that as sleep arises and the abdomen becomes warmer, all the airy material leaves the veins, and death ensues.

In the collection of multi-authored case notes known as The Epidemics, Hippocratic authors discuss matters of sleep and related symptoms. They believed that in sleep, blood retreats further into the interior. We now understand that sleep involves blood redistribution, supporting this belief.

The Hippocratic text, 'On Breaths', wrongly emphasises the effects of cooling of the blood on sleep, and air as responsible for illness. The body does, of course, usually cool during sleep.

Aphorisms 2. III, states:

Sleep, insomnia, either happening more than normal measure, is bad.

Ὕπνος, ἀγρυπνίη, ἀμφότερα μᾶλλον τοῦ μετρίου γινόμενα, κακόν.

In the Coan Prenotions 487, there is a prescription for sleep hygiene:

'The best way to sleep is how one is accustomed to whenever healthy; but to lie on one's back, with legs stretched out, is not good. If he [the patient] sinks down in bed towards the foot, it is very bad. It is fatal to yawn and always sleep, and for the legs of someone sleeping on their back to be forcefully bent together and twisted. To lie on the stomach if not accustomed to, signals derangement and pains in the

abdomen. To have the feet and hands uncovered, when not strongly heated, and to kick around the legs, is bad, for it signals anguish. To want to sit up is bad in acute cases, and the worst in pneumonias and pleurisies. One should sleep at night, and be awake during the day. The opposite is grievous. It would be least harmful to sleep from dawn to the first third of the day; those who sleep after this are in a sorry way. Worst is to sleep neither in the day nor at night, for if he is kept awake by bodily pain and distress, he will be deranged because of this sign. For the Hippocratic physician, a good regimen is the foundation for maintaining health, since it can be affected so easily by the foods eaten, drinks consumed, exercise taken and, as is evident from the above accounts, the patterns of sleep.'

Several observations in this passage are pertinent to TFE symptoms:

- 'To kick around the legs, is bad, for it signals anguish.'
- 'To want to sit up is bad in acute cases, and the worst in pneumonias and pleurisies.'
- 'One should sleep at night, and be awake during the day. The opposite is grievous.'
- 'Worst is to sleep neither in the day nor at night.'

We can agree that both agitated REM sleep and sleep deprivation are not beneficial, whereas following the normal sleep-wake circadian rhythm, is healthy. Modern physicians differ in thinking that the sitting position will benefit the breathing of cases with pneumonia and pleurisy.

Psukhē 'On Regimen IV' highlights the importance of sleep:

'For while the sleeping body does not perceive, the awakened soul knows all things – it sees that which is visible, hears that which is audible, walks, touches, is distressed, reflects. In short, as many as the services of the body or of the soul, all such things the soul effects for itself in sleep.'

'On Regimen' also mentions the effect of stress on sleep: 'Just as in the waking state the face is flushed and the eyes are bloodshot, whenever he is afraid, and his intelligence conceives of something bad being done, so too he suffers in sleep.'

People believed that Asclepius cured the sick while they slept. In the case of Agameda of Ceos: 'She slept in the Temple for offspring and saw a dream. It seemed to her in her sleep that a serpent lay on her belly. And thereupon five children were born to her.'

From the fifth century BC, the serpent became prominent in Asclepian iconography. The relationship between the serpent and the god was multifaceted: the snake being used as a symbol, an avatar, an embodiment, or even a pet.

Asclepius was, however, 'quick to reverse the cure he has bestowed, should he not be properly honoured':

'Hermon of Thasus. His blindness was cured by Asclepius. But since afterwards he did not bring the thank-offerings, the god made him blind again. When he came back and slept in the Temple again, [the god] made him well.'

The fourth book of the Hippocratic 'On Regimen' comprises a Greek dream book. It provides a guide to interpreting the various symbols or encounters one might experience in dreams:

Περὶ δὲ τῶν τεκμηρίων τῶν ἐν τοῖσιν ὕπνοισιν ὅστις ὀρθῶς ἔγνωκε, μεγάλην ἔχοντα δύναμιν εὑρήσει πρὸς ἅπαντα.

'Whoever has correctly learnt about the sure signs happening in sleep, will discover that they have a great influence upon all things.' Also:

ὅστις οὖν ἐπίσταται κρίνειν ταῦτα ὀρθῶς μέγα μέρος ἐπίσταται σοφίης.

'Whoever, then, is acquainted with interpreting these things correctly, is acquainted with a great part of wisdom'.

This type of prognostic work evidently bears a fundamental similarity to divination.

In 'Day Residue' Dreams, it states:

'Such dreams as render in the night the very actions or thoughts of men during the day, coming to pass according to habit – just as were carried out or deliberated on during the day already in genuine actions – these things for man are good. For this signifies health, because the soul abides by the purposes of the day, and is mastered neither by surfeit or depletion, nor by any other matter attacking from the outside.'

In 'of dreams', in 'On Regimen', the Hippocratic author considers imagery that involves the natural environment and the individual reaction to it:

'To clearly see and clearly hear those things upon the earth, to run without faltering and walk without faltering, quickly, without fear, to see the earth smooth and well tilled, and flourishing trees with much fruit and cultivated, and flowing rivers on their course, and pure water neither higher nor lower than is fitting, and springs and wells the same; all of these things signify health to the individual.'

For Lucretius, dreams were not to be feared, given they have no real import. (Magowan, S.R. 2017).

In 2000 BCE, people would advertise themselves as professional dream interpreters, preceding Sigmund Freud by 4000 years (Freud, S. 1901).

Authors have mentioned sleep throughout literature; in the Old Testament, Jacob dreamed of a ladder reaching Heaven, and Joseph interpreted the dreams of the Egyptian Pharaoh.

Shakespeare mentions sleep:

To sleep: perchance to dream: ay, there's the rub; For in that sleep of death what dreams may come.

Hamlet, Act 3, Scene 1

Sleep that knits up the ravell'd sleave of care, The death of each day's life, sore labour's bath, Balm of hurt minds, great nature's second course, Chief nourisher in life's feast.

Macbeth, Act 2, Scene 2

More modern writers have not ignored sleep:

What, but thee Sleep? Soft closer of our eyes! Low murmurer of tender lullabies!

John Keats. Sleep and Poetry.

It appears that every man's insomnia is as different from his neighbor's as are their daytime hopes and aspirations.

The Crack-Up, 'Sleeping and Waking'

F. Scott Fitzgerald.

Both sculpture and painting often depict sleep. From Renaissance art, through to Impressionist paintings, sleeping figures are a frequent subject. Sleeping figures alone, and those shown with wakeful figures, illustrate the vulnerability of sleep and the suspension of reasoning. A question often posed is whether the subject is dead or sleeping. Time appears stopped, both in sleep and in death.

In Sandro Botticelli's Mars and Venus, the clothed Venus sits upright and alert, while sleeping Mars lies incapacitated and vulnerable. Venus appears in control, while baby satyrs use Mars as a play-thing.

In his 1891 oil painting of 'The Doctor', Luke Fildes portrays a family doctor patiently waiting with the parents for the recovery of their sick sleeping child. Will she wake or die? Is sleep curative or just a feature of illness? The painting leaves the question unanswered. If she survives the crisis (of pneumonia, perhaps), she should live.

An interest in sleep has no cultural boundaries. The states of waking, dreaming, and deep sleep are associated with the syllable 'aum' that Hindus chant when they meditate.

In the early 20th century, both Sigmund Freud, and Carl Jung were interested in the significance of dreams.

'We also live in our dreams, we do not live only by day. Sometimes we accomplish our greatest deeds in dreams.'

Carl G. Jung. The Red Book.

'The dream is a spontaneous self-portrayal, in symbolic form, of the actual situation in the unconscious ... The dream is specifically the utterance of the unconscious.'

Carl G. Jung: Structure and Dynamics of the Psyche.

'According to Sigmund Freud (1900), sources of dreams include stimuli from the external world, subjective experiences, organic stimuli within the body, and mental activities during sleep.' These assertions have some support from empirical evidence (Zhang, W., Guo, B. 2018).

The current theory is that dreaming allows self-organisation. It posits that, 'memory consolidation, emotion regulation, and reception of external stimuli can contribute to dream content

(Zhang, W. 2016); hence, dream content can contain important information about the dreamer.' (Zhang, W., Guo. B. 2018).

CHAPTER SIX

The Role of Sleep, and Sleep Disturbance in TFE

'And sleep that sometime shuts up sorrow's eye,
Steal me awhile from mine own company.'

Helena.
A Midsummer Night's Dream.

Many molecules regulate sleep and arousal, with cholinergic and other neurons playing an important role in the sleep regulation of mammals.

Both circadian and homeostatic mechanisms are involved in sleep regulation. The circadian clock controls the timing of sleep, and the homeostatic mechanism controls the sleep drive. The latter is less understood than circadian rhythm.

Many patients with TFE symptoms notice a sleep paradox. The more tired they are, the less well they sleep. This is usually conditional on sleep being disturbed by continuing stress, especially those involving fear, unresolved decisions, and pending situations. The sleep they get has been called paradoxical sleep.

Stress disturbs normal sleep, but so do some drugs, mental and physical illness. Febrile illness, psychiatric conditions like depression or mania, and painful conditions like toothache, arthritis, and neuralgia can all affect it. Stimulatory drugs, like cocaine and amphetamine, can cause sleep deprivation.

Effective and Ineffective Sleep

In hibernating animals, like the arctic snow fox, the activity of astrocytes and microglia becomes attenuated. This is associated with reduced EEG power spectra. (Zhou, F. et al. 2001). Hibernation reduces power spectra beyond levels seen in normal human NREM sleep. One function of sleep is thus power conservation. In hibernation, occasional wakeful periods occur, and episodic respiration is seen, similar to that of human sleep apnoea (Kildulf, T.S. et al. 1993).

The human body cycles through two phases of sleep: rapid eye movement (REM) sleep, and non-rapid eye movement (NREM) sleep. NREM sleep has been further divided into three stages: N1 to N3. Each phase and stage of sleep exhibits variations in muscle tone, brain wave pattern, and eye movement. The body cycles through all stages, 4 to 6 times each night, averaging 90 minutes for each cycle (Memar, P. et al. 2018).

Jet lag and shift work cause tiredness by advancing or delaying the sleep phase.

In delayed sleep phase syndrome (DSPS), subjects find it difficult to fall asleep and wake up. DSPS can cause severe daytime sleepiness, with changes in mood and behaviour. Disturbed sleep, sleep apnoea, sedative medication, some psychiatric conditions, and sleep disorders like narcolepsy also cause daytime sleepiness.

The third and fourth phases of sleep, being more restful, have long been thought to be restorative. Newer information has associated them with memory and learning. During these phases, tissue growth, and repair take place, important hormones are released, and cellular energy restored (Patel, A.K. et al. 2024).

Sleep quality and time spent in each sleep stage is altered by depression, aging, traumatic brain injuries, medications, and circadian rhythm disorders.

In the brain, gamma-aminobutyric acid (GABA) is a primary inhibitory transmitter. When GABA is bound to GABA-A receptors, sleep is induced (Gottesmann, C. 2012). Sleep-promoting areas in the anterior hypothalamus release GABA. GABA also inhibits wake-promoting areas in the hypothalamus and brainstem (Murillo-Rodriguez, E., et al. 2009). Adenosine can also promote sleep by inhibiting areas in the basal forebrain (Watson, C.J. et al. 2010).

Most cortical acetylcholine ACh is released during waking and REM sleep. It is lowest during NREM sleep (Vazquez, J. 2001). Acetylcholine (ACh), dopamine, norepinephrine (NE), serotonin, histamine, and the hypocretin peptides work together to maintain the waking state. Noradrenergic cells inhibit REM sleep and promote wakefulness. Other brain areas are involved in arousal: the thalamus, hypothalamus, basal forebrain, and cortex.

Sleep duration gets shorter with age. Those over 65-years of age, sleep 1.5 hours less on average than those 18-years old. (Chaput, J.P. 2020).

A circadian rhythm controls both sleep and the nocturnal release of adrenocorticotropic hormone (ACTH), prolactin, and NE.

The physiological functions of sleep have been the subject of much research. Apart from being restorative of mental energy, sleep facilitates neural maturation, learning, and memory. During sleep, clearance of metabolic waste products, and the conservation of metabolic energy occur (Frank, M.,G. 2019).

Phases of 'Normal' Sleep

The clinical evaluation of sleep uses polysomnography, a procedure that utilises an electroencephalogram (EEG), the electro-oculogram, electromyogram, electrocardiogram, pulse oximetry, airflow, and respiratory effort.

We spend 75% of sleep in the NREM stages. A typical night's sleep comprises 4 to 5 sleep cycles, with a complete sleep cycle taking between one and a half to two hours. The first REM period is short, and as the night progresses, longer periods of REM and decreased time in deep sleep (NREM) occur.

During wakefulness, EEG recordings show beta waves of high frequency and low amplitude. One can observe alpha waves during quiet/relaxed wakefulness. Both depend on whether the eyes are open or closed.

The first stage of sleep is the wake, or W stage, which further depends on whether the eyes are open or closed. During eye-open wakefulness, beta waves predominate. Alpha waves become the predominant pattern, as individuals become drowsy and close their eyes.

During light sleep (N1 phase; 5% of sleep), EEGs record low voltage theta waves, muscle tone is maintained, and breathing is regular. This stage lasts 1 to 5 minutes.

During deeper sleep (N2: 45% of total sleep), lasting 25 minutes in the first cycle. N2 lengthens in subsequent cycles, with sleep spindles and K complexes (long delta waves—low frequency, high amplitude). Sleep spindles are brief, powerful bursts of neuronal firing in the superior temporal gyri, etc. Heart rate and body temperature drop. Memory consolidation, would seem to depend on sleep spindles, while maintaining sleep depends on K-complexes.

In the deepest sleep phase, (N3), low-frequency delta waves appear (25% of NREM sleep). This is known as slow-wave sleep (SWS). During this phase, waking the subject is most difficult. Aging reduces the time spent in this slow, delta-wave sleep, increasing the time spent in N2 sleep. If woken during this stage, mental fogginess (sleep inertia) occurs. This is characterised by moderately impaired mental performance, lasting 30 to 60 minutes (Hilditch, C.J. 2019). In this phase, the body builds bone and muscle, and immune changes occur. Sleepwalking, night terrors, and bedwetting can also happen.

During REM sleep, beta-waves similar to those of wakefulness appear on EEG. REM is associated with dreaming and nightmares.

It is not restful. During these phases, skeletal muscles are atonic, except for the eyes and diaphragmatic muscles, which remain active. Breathing rate becomes erratic. Starting 90 minutes after sleep starts, REM cycles become longer throughout the night. The first cycle usually lasts 10 minutes, and the last cycle is up to one hour.

During REM phases, increased oxygen consumption occurs (sometimes increasing by >20%). Increased synthesis of cerebral ACh occurs, and the heart rate increases (Peever, J. 2017). Fig. 3 presents a schematic diagram of energy expenditure during waking and sleep periods.

Disturbances of Normal Sleep

Loss of sleep causes an increase in sleep drive, with deficits in hippocampal-dependent memory. Both responses require activation of adenosine A1 receptors (adorA1Rs) and the release of transmitter molecules which include ATP. Astrocyte ATP is rapidly converted to adenosine in the extracellular space, in a process termed gliotransmission.' (Schmitt, L.I. et al. 2012).

Schmitt,L.I. et al., showed that the level of adorA1R activation increases in response to wakefulness in mice (Mus musculus). This increase affects synaptic transmission in the hippocampus and modulates network activity in the cortex. The net extracellular concentration of ATP increases in response to normal wakefulness and sleep deprivation. Wakefulness increases the level of extracellular adenosine in the hippocampus, together with the release of transmitters from astrocytes. Astrocytes modulate the accumulation of sleep drive and its cognitive consequences through a pathway involving A1 receptors (Halassa, M.M. et al. 2009).

Sleep Apnoea

With obstructed breathing, reduced time in both N3 and REM sleep occurs. Hypoxia, cardiac dysrhythmias, and death can occur. As a result, excessive daytime drowsiness is common. Two sleep apnoea types exist: central and obstructive. In central sleep apnoea, the brain cannot signal respiratory muscles. Obstructive sleep apnoea is mechanical, leading to a partial or complete blockage of the upper airway (Labarca, G. et al. 2018).

There is no benefit in hypercapnia, except that it renders sleep induction easy, the price of which is permanent somnolence. Charles Dickens gives an example of a young boy with Obesity Hypoventilation Syndrome (Pickwick Papers, 1837):

"Sleep!" said the old gentleman, 'he's always asleep. Goes on errands fast asleep, and snores as he waits at table."
"How very odd!" said Mr. Pickwick.
"Ah! odd indeed," returned the old gentleman; "I'm proud of that boy–wouldn't part with him on any account–he's a natural curiosity!"

REM Sleep Disorder

During REM sleep, the usual muscle atonia can be lost, and dreams with vocalisation and sudden limb movements can occur. Sometimes seen in Parkinson's disease, and Lewy body dementia, it can be associated with antidepressant use.

Narcolepsy

Narcolepsy causes persistent daytime sleepiness and brief episodes of muscle weakness (cataplexy). Individuals can skip the initial phases of sleep and straightaway enter REM sleep. Patients can dream during brief naps, and become atonic and paralysed for periods lasting seconds to minutes, at any time of day.

Somnambulism

Sleepwalking, or somnambulism, occurs during N3 and REM sleep in school-aged children. They are not acting out their dreams because in REM sleep, muscles are paralysed. Activities like dressing, eating, and urinating can occur.

Depression

Patients with depression can have increased total REM sleep, and a decrease in the interval between sleep onset and the start of the first REM period (Steiger, A. 2019). Disturbed sleep and early morning wakening are both typical features of depression and chronic fatigue. The monoamine deficiency theory suggests that in depression, there is a depletion of neurotransmitters serotonin, nor-epinephrine and dopamine. This can be seen in the mid-brain and brainstem nuclei, together with their radiations to other areas. Any pharmaceutical that increases the amounts of these transmitters can improve depression (Hasler, G. 2010).

The EEG in depression has some specific characteristics (elevated alpha and beta-2 activity in the pre-frontal cortex; elevated beta-3 in the medial occipital cortex (Liu, X. et al. 2024). Also observed is a more random network structure and increased signal complexity. The imaging of the brain in depression exhibits significant variation. Its non-replication makes it of little use in clinical diagnosis (Dunlop, B.W. & Mayberg, H.S. 2017).

Many patients with TFE symptoms are clinically depressed, so to what extent is their neurophysiology similar? In sleep deprivation, adenosine levels increase and inhibit neural activity. Inhibition of cholinergic nuclei can also be pronounced. The decrease in cortical acetylcholine seems to cause the effect of sleep deprivation. Most research studies focus on short-term sleep deprivation and the resulting tiredness. This tiredness is usually relieved by one or two nights of normal sleep. In clinical practice, long-term disturbed sleep causes TFE symptoms, and a few night's sleep will not readily restore normal cerebral functioning (attention, executive behaviour, verbal fluency, etc.). During the recovery phase of sleep deprivation, marked slow theta-wave sleep can occur. Imaging studies suggest a reduction in pre-frontal cortical activity, with considerable variation seen between subjects, sometimes resembling the changes associated with aging (Boonstra, T.W. et al. 2007).

The effect of long-term disturbed sleep remains poorly understood. In the short-term, there would seem to be many neurotransmitter differences distinguishing depression from the tiredness and fatigue that follow short-term sleep deprivation. Long-term sleep deprivation has, however, remained unstudied, even though TFE symptoms are common.

Ageing

About 43% of older individuals, have difficulty with sleep initiation. Insomnia and earlier wake times also occur (Ancoli-Israel, S. 2000). Many studies have suggested it is the advancing of circadian rhythm accompanying age that causes irregular melatonin and cortisol secretion. Older individuals sleep 36% less than children aged 5-years. While the ability to sleep becomes more difficult with age, the need for sleep does not decrease. Night-time wakening, nocturia, and decreased mobility may be associated. A progressive decrease in time spent in slow wave sleep can occur.

Traumatic Brain Injury

Traumatic brain injury patients can experience prolonged sleep onset, shorter total sleep times, and more waking at night than controls. They spend less time in REM sleep. These individuals report poor sleep quality, more daytime dysfunction, and the use of more sleep medication (Aoun, R. 2019).

The Causes of Disturbed Sleep

Intermittent nocturnal hypoxia, sleep fragmentation and autonomic dysregulation, can all cause sleep disturbance. Sleepiness is commoner amongst those reporting depression or anxiety disorders, since it affects their quality of life (Slater, G., Steier, J. 2012). In my experience, it's the continuous presence of unresolved problems, especially those that threaten security and the maintenance of lifestyle, that have the most impact on sleep.

Sleep Disorder Epidemiology

Sleep disorders are now grouped into six major categories in the ICSD-3-TR (The AASM International Classification of Sleep Disorders – Third. The American Academy of Sleep Medicine):

- Insomnia Disorders.
- Sleep-Related Breathing Disorders.
- Central Disorders of Hypersomnolence.
- Circadian Rhythm Sleep-Wake Disorders.
- Parasomnia.
- Sleep-Related Movement Disorders.

Daytime sleepiness, caused by disturbed sleep, can be debilitating and dangerous, with possible medico-legal implications.

Being involved in concerning situations can disturb sleep and cause daytime tiredness. Clinicians may choose to overlook these situations, with not all circumstances being stressful. They can relate to pleasurable but unresolved issues: whether to marry; whether to go to college; how to invest inherited money. Sleep can process questions, sometimes yielding satisfactory answers upon waking.

The "Sleep in America" poll, conducted in 2008 by the American Sleep Foundation, found 18% of respondents scoring ten points or more on the Epworth Sleepiness Score (ESS), categorised as 'excessively sleepy'. (Swanson, L.M. et al. 2011).

A Japanese study asked whether subjects had ever fallen asleep when inadvisable (when driving a car). A prevalence of 2.5% was found (Kaneita, Y. et al. 2005).

A Norwegian study in which the ESS was administered by telephone, found 17.7% of participants with an ESS score of 10 or more (Pallesen, S. et al. (2007). A US study, assessed daytime sleepiness by asking, "do you feel drowsy or sleepy most of the day, but manage to stay awake?" and, "do you have any irresistible sleep attacks during the day?", found a prevalence of 8.7% (Bixler, E.O. et al. 2005).

In a sleep survey of adults in Finland, Hublin, C. et al. (1996) asked about sleepiness during the day: snoring and disordered breathing; insomnia (sleeplessness); depression; use of tranquillisers; insufficient sleep and narcolepsy. Nine per-cent had daytime sleepiness (66% of whom were women). The occurrence of sleepiness decreased with age, and was unaffected by BMI, shift work, or coffee consumption. Alcohol and smoking were associated with more daytime sleepiness.

Eleven per-cent of women and 6.7% of men noticed daytime sleepiness every day. Of those who were tired, 25% were thought depressed, with attendant sleep problems (early morning waking and poor quality sleep). Nine per-cent had too little time for sleep, while 20.7% of women and 28.6% of men complained of insomnia at least every other night. Sleep upset, related to breathing difficulties, was caused by lung disorders or obesity, and associated with snoring and other forms of respiratory obstruction. These occurred in 19.5% of women and 42.3% of men.

Poor night time sleep does not always predict daytime sleepiness, whether judged by the reports of insomniacs, or confirmed in a sleep laboratory (Lichstein, et al. 1994). They compared only 20 insomniacs with 20 non-insomniacs. With a lack of statistical power, perhaps their results can only reflect the variance of energy available to different individuals during the day, and individual differences in the effectiveness of sleep.

TFE from sleep disturbance can have important clinical associations. Ford and Kamerow (1989) noted the prevalence of sleep disturbance in a community (10.2% had insomnia; 3.2% hypersomnia). They found that 40% of those with insomnia, and 46.5% of those with hypersomnia, had a psychiatric problem (compared to 16.5% in controls). When followed for one year, those with an unabated sleep problem were much more likely to develop a psychiatric problem (odds ratio: 39.8). It was less for those whose sleep disturbance had abated during the one-year follow-up period (odds ratio: 1.6).

Partinen, M. et al. (1984) enquired about insomnia in different work groups. Male labourers complained most; 28.1% waking at least three times at night. The number for male physicians was 4.9%. Heart attacks are more common in the unskilled labour force, the group in which insomnia (but not hypersomnia) is most common (13.4%, compared to 8% in executives). This difference is worthy of discussion, since it may in part account for the health divide (Bambra, Claire. 2016).

The link between shift work, sleep and cardiovascular disease might be explained by a mismatch of circadian rhythms, social disruption, and other stresses.

The odds of insomnia decrease as the number of employees increases. Mostly, the prevalence of insomnia is highest in workplaces with less than five employees (Lee, J. et al. 2021).

Researchers exposed subjects to the heat of a sauna to investigate the mechanism through which stress might affect the cardiovascular system. What resulted was an increase in plasma adrenaline with no change in noradrenaline, free fatty acid, or triglyceride concentrations. Emotional stress, by contrast, is associated with the release of free fatty acids and hyper-triglyceridaemia, both risk factors for the development of atheroma (Taggart, P. et al. 1972).

In an early study, Friedman, M. et al. (1958), studied the effect of work stress on CVS blood risk factors. The highest serum cholesterol and clotting acceleration occurred during severe occupational or other stress. They were lowest during minimal stress.

Work stress affects sleep, and sleep can affect the outcomes of CVS disease. The relationship between work stress and CVS disease was the subject of the landmark Whitehall Studies (Bosma, H., et al. 1998), under the direction of Michael Marmot.

They postulated two alternative job stress models: high status, low job strain; low status, high job strain. 'Women reported high effort and low reward conditions more often than men (48% and 41%, respectively). Moreover, men and women in lower employment grades reported effort-reward imbalance more often than subjects in higher grades.' In those with lower status, a higher prevalence of hostility, a blocked career, and poor promotion prospects were prevalent. Higher status individuals experienced work-related over-commitment and competitiveness.

They found the lowest prevalence of job strain in the highest employment grades. Job demands were also highest in the higher grades, reported by 45%, compared with 10% in the lowest grade levels.

They showed effort-reward imbalance associated with elevated risks of subsequent coronary heart disease. 'The risk of coronary heart disease for men and women who have both high efforts and low rewards, is about three times as high as that for subjects with low efforts and high rewards (ORs varied from 2.59 to 3.63)'.

New coronary heart disease was not universally related to job strain. Only self-reported job strain and coronary heart disease in men were associated (Odds Ratio [OR]: 1.45). No correlation was found between job demands and job control, although low job control was found consistently related to new coronary heart disease reports. Differences in gender, effort-reward imbalance or job control were not statistically significant. Both effort-reward imbalance and low job control have strong and significant associations with the coronary heart disease outcomes in the total sample. 'Odds ratios of any coronary heart disease outcome were 3.14, 2.04, and 1.57, for effort-reward imbalance (high efforts and low rewards), self-reported low job control, and externally assessed low job control, respectively.'

In another study of women at work, Haynes, S.G. et al. (1980), found that more women than men reported symptoms of emotional distress. 'Working women and men were more likely to report Type A behaviour, ambitiousness, and marital disagreements than were housewives. Working women experienced more job mobility than men, and more daily stress and marital dissatisfaction than housewives or men.' Working women did not have significantly higher incidence rates of CHD than housewives (7.8 vs 5.4 per cent, respectively), but those holding clerical jobs had double the CHD rate of housewives. Many clerical workers had suppressed hostility, a non-supportive boss, and decreased job mobility. CHD rates were highest among working women who had married, and who had raised three or more children. Among working women, clerical workers who had children and were married to blue-collar workers had the highest risk of CHD (21.3 %). In the latter studies, work stress and insomnia are correlation to CHD, but TFE symptoms received no mention.

It is said that insomnia is a state of conditioned hyperarousal (Riemann, D. 2010). It is defined by the American Academy of Sleep Medicine as 'a perceived difficulty with sleep initiation, consolidation, duration, or quality, despite an adequate opportunity to sleep, coupled with subsequent daytime impairment, and as chronic when lasting at least 3 months' (Edinger, J.D., et al. 2004).

Insomnia has been associated with an inflammatory response (Irwin, M.R. 2015), greater atherogenesis (King, C.R. et al. 2008)(Meier-Ewert, H.K. et al. 2004), involvement of the hypothalamic-pituitary axis (increased cortisol levels)(Rodenbeck, A. et al. 2003), the sympathetic nervous system, and increased insulin resistance.

In a review of studies linking insomnia with short sleep duration and cardiovascular problems (hypertension, coronary artery disease, and heart failure), an increased risk of hypertension, acute coronary syndrome, and heart failure has been found (Partinen, M., et al. 1982)(Javaheri, S. Redline, S. 2017).

The symptoms noted, were reduced attention, concentration, and memory; fatigue, and energy reduction; accidents at work and while driving; daytime sleepiness, mood disturbances, and irritability. One feature was specifically worrying about sleep. A higher prevalence of heart attacks, was found in those who sleep more than nine hours on average, with angina commoner than expected in those who sleep less than six hours, and those who sleep over ten hours (Partinen, M. et al. 1982). Long sleep is associated with more REM sleep: sleep known to stimulate the heart and circulation. Those with respiratory disorders get more tired, sleep longer, and have a higher prevalence of heart attacks during sleep.

Clinical Significance of Disturbed Sleep

We all spend two-thirds of our lives asleep. Between 50 and 70 million Americans report sleep difficulties. Lack of sleep affects our memory and ability to think. Sleep deprivation can lead to a poorer quality of life and well-being, neurological dysfunction, mood swings, hallucinations, and poor executive functioning. Those who do not get enough sleep are at higher risk of accidents, and of developing obesity, diabetes, and cardiovascular disease (Institute of Medicine, US. 2006).

Difficulty falling or staying asleep (insomnia), despite the opportunity for sleep, is associated with impaired daytime functioning in about 10% of people. Many treatments have been used. They include sleep hygiene (reducing light and noise), cognitive behavioural therapy (CBT), and various pharmacological therapies: benzodiazepines, melatonin receptor agonists, selective histamine antagonists, antidepressants, antipsychotics, anticonvulsants, and non-selective antihistamines.

Alcohol and benzodiazepines can cause decreased REM sleep. Benzodiazepines are a significant class of drugs used for insomnia. They can increase the arousal threshold and decrease the overall time spent in stage N3 and REM sleep. They can be useful, however, in reducing night terrors and sleepwalking, occurring most in the N3 and REM sleep phases (Holbrook, A. 2001).

The more severe the TFE symptoms, the greater the inability to sleep. This sleep paradox drives the progression of TFE symptoms towards exhaustion; a frequent forerunner of ill-health and the progression of some medical conditions.

In my clinical experience, few cope well with daytime problems, unless they have sufficient untroubled sleep. Perhaps those who can lack anxiety or enough dedicated involvement. They might escape the sleep paradox that so often defeats those distressed by life's problems.

The process of adapting to de-stabilising physiological influences that could disturb the milieu intérieur, like dehydration, heat, cold, acidic and salty food, etc., was propounded by the French physiologist Claude Bernard (1813-1878). Sleep holds an important place in the process. He showed that organs like the liver can have multiple functions, and that some metabolic processes exhibit reversibility (like the conversion of glycogen to glucose). He also proposed that adaptive bodily processes attempt to keep the status quo (homeostasis), but will fail if the disturbing factors are too strong to overcome.

Bernard proposed experimental medicine. At the end of the 20th century, the acronym OPHERIC was given to Bernard's hypothetico-deductive approach: first, make an Observation which poses a Problem (a question). Then formulate a Hypothesis that claims to solve the problem. Then, design and carry out an Experiment, to invalidate or confirm the hypothesis. The Results of this experiment are collected and Interpreted to draw a Conclusion. Of course, every discovery opens new questions; 'this is how medical science always progresses today'. (Habert, R. 2022).

Without sleep, daytime tiredness will progress through fatigue to exhaustion, and the risk of a sudden catastrophic clinical event increases. Like all cliff-edge catastrophic phenomena, only a small extra stimulus is required to bring about major change (Thom, René, 1972. mathematical topologist); the situation is thus bi-stable: from a body intact to one fractured; from stable arterial plaque with some platelet adhesion, to occluding clot formation and possible infarction.

Sleep Management

Humans cannot cope without sleep. Restful sleep refreshes those who become tired of toiling with life. While some sleep is recuperative, disturbed sleep often results in daytime tiredness. Fast heart rates, high blood pressure, and daytime levels of physiological activity can accompany dreaming during REM sleep. REM sleep is an active dreaming state of disputed function, not a restful state (Fig. 3).

Freud believed dreams to be glimpses into the workings of our sub-conscious. The significance of dreams has remained controversial, with no means of verifying any theory. Some believe that dreams help to anticipate how we might cope with future events. They may need repeating if they fail to acknowledge a solution or fail to confirm our coping ability. Jung thought dreams represented a conversation between our self and ego. Freud disputed this, believing dreams to be fantasy, lies, and distortions of the truth. A more modern view is that dreaming consolidates our memories of the day.

In 1953, Hall first suggested that dreams expressed ourselves in relation to those who co-exist in our environment (Hall, C. 1971). More recently, Erik Hoel expressed the view that dreams are disruptive, allowing our reasoning to become unstuck. Fictional narratives and art can be disruptive influences, perhaps inciting lateral thinking and finding solutions to problems difficult to solve. He links dreaming to creativity. This might explain why we can go to sleep with a problem, and wake with a solution. Birds and mammals dream, but reptiles do not. Reptiles are pre-programmed to survive without a mother's help; mammals and birds must go through a learning process with rumination in dreams to help survival (Hoel, E. 2021).

Regardless of any dream theory, REM sleep consumes more energy than it replenishes (Fig. 3).

Sleep induction works best when we control the prevailing conditions. Repetitive motion or a boring environment can help. A slow relaxing experience, under conditions of reduced light and noise, aide sleep induction. Disturbing and challenging entertainment or arguments before sleep can inhibit induction. Sleep induction disorders occur in those troubled by pain, restlessness, and psychiatric conditions, any of which may increase arousal. Optimal sleep conditions vary, ranging from those who can sleep anywhere to those with stringent requirements (Kandola, A. 2024).

Optimal sleep induction will benefit from time-clock considerations, especially after long-haul flights. Circadian rhythm and the production of melatonin are important considerations, although no official recommendation yet exists, for taking melatonin to enable sleep (Costello, R.B. et al. 2014).

The Biological Clock

Throughout each 24-hour cycle of sleep, wakefulness, hormones, body temperature, alertness, and sleepiness follow an internal body clock, driven by the pineal hormone melatonin. This 'clock' is driven by daylight. Without light exposure, and no knowledge of day or night-time, the cycle length can vary between 25 and 27-hours, with peaks and troughs that are different for each of us (Mills, J.N. et al. 1974). For most, alertness and executive efficiency, is maximal in the morning, when most business is done. For rarer, 'evening people', alertness comes at the end of the usual working (for most others): between 5 to 9 pm. So called 'night people', peak between 12 midnight to 4 a.m. Such people are rare. In over 50-years of medical practice, I recognised only two.

Alcohol, Food, and Sleep

Some patients believe that a meal before sleep will cause wakefulness. However, most find that food promotes sleep. This may be the effect of blood fat, lowered hormone levels, increased cytokines, like IL-1 (Lehrskov, L.L. et al. 2018), the induction of cerebral slow waves, or the effect of foods containing melatonin. Meals can induce palpitation and increase arousal, while others might suffer indigestion from a peptic ulcer; acid regurgitation and heartburn from a hiatus hernia (on lying down). They will benefit from an early meal and medication (such as an antacid, proton pump inhibitor or histamine H2-receptor antagonist). Alcohol can disturb sleep and affect mental and physical functioning.

Alcohol can affect sleep in a complicated and perverse way, although advised for sleep induction for millennia. Many depend on it for sedated sleep. While small amounts can create an optimum level of sedation, too much can cause agitation and deny effective sleep. Alcohol both stimulates and suppresses the brain. It is responsible for changes in sleep architecture: more REM sleep, and effects on slow-wave sleep (Colrain, I.M. et al. 2014). The effect of alcohol on the brain lasts longer than a few hours. Its effect on arousal, from a disturbing mixture of stimulation and sedation, can impair well-being and performance. This has important economic consequences.

A few decades ago, in the City of London, a significant number of office managers did little work after lunch because of alcohol intake. Alcohol impairs the performance of drivers and pilots. Slowed reaction times can follow alcohol induced sleep deprivation. Tiredness and debilitating illness can produce similar effects.

For moderate drinkers, a revelation awaits. Abstinence often allows more restful sleep and improved daytime energy. In times of stress, drinking alcohol can improve relaxation, and seem to help one cope. Excessive alcohol intake will deteriorate performance, but can be mis-perceived as helpful. Problem solving is most helped by alcohol abstinence in the longer term.

Sleep Surrogates

Resting in a quasi-sleep state, while lying on a beach or meditating, will reduce the energy spent on cognition and emotive thought. People often assume (within the canon of world literature) that sleep, relaxation, and less talking are beneficial.

Many and various views about preserving our energy abound in media publications. For instance, 'Every time we open our mouths we release a powerful energy. If we could learn to hold on to that energy, it could be used to nurture our dreams, heal our bodies and fuel our minds.' Also, 'Talking is something we must learn to use, not something we must always do. There is a power in silence that energises the mind, body and soul.' 'When we perfect the art of silence, chances are we will get a lot more done.' (Vazant, I. 1995).

Scientific support for the clinical benefits of energy-reducing behaviour is lacking. Nobody has yet proved that those who relax, sleep well, or talk less, will live longer or suffer fewer illnesses. These are likely to be mere ripples, superimposed on what are the tsunami strength effects on morbidity and mortality caused by genetic makeup.

There can be little doubt that those who suffer illness seem to recover faster when able to sleep. The beneficial changes for wounded soldiers, observed by Florence Nightingale during the Crimean War, support the view that sleep aids healing. The science of immunity has been slow to support her observations. (Segerstrom, S.C. & Miller, G.E. 2004).

Buddhism, in recognising the place of personal pain and suffering, can reduce energy expenditure by denying the need for ego and avarice. It prescribes meditation, to dispense with energy waste, and to achieve harmony, contentment, tranquillity, composure, and peace within. Living for the moment, with no need for analysis, decision making, planning or prediction, will reduce mental energy expenditure. The many life consequences of mindless behaviour, however, are another matter.

Westerners may find it easy to criticise Buddhist attitudes. While meditating beneath a bodhi tree can be beneficial, for most westerners, it will be more difficult to achieve composure in the workplace or during inter-personal conflict. The rejoinder is that Buddhist's neither work in offices, nor engage in conflicting relationships.

The Sabbath and Biological Function

The fast erosion of the Sabbath from the lives of non-practising Christians and Jews, caused by 24-hour, seven-day working and shopping, night-shifts, and entertainment, has meant the loss of valuable time for relaxation, and restful mindfulness. Even education has succumbed.

The head teacher at a comprehensive school in Great Horton, once said: *"The youngster have a tremendous thirst for work, and when I offered them the Sunday morning classes they nearly bit my hand off... We are trying to tap into their motivation; and for them to come in on Sundays affirms the strength within themselves to do well."*

The Times,
16th December 1996.

Religious conviction is necessary to appreciate the health significance of the Sabbath; a day of rest, or a weekly change in usual activity. Change in routine can be refreshing, and an afternoon sleep recharging. While those with a religious faith spend their Sabbath in reflection, prayer, and spiritual refreshment, they might also tap into the self-esteem that rewards the dutiful and the observant. Solace and comfort can, however, also be found in non-religious ritual.

Time off improves health and well-being. It provides people, usually busy with worldly pursuits, to spend time together; time with their families and friends, practising the piano or reading the evermore voluminous Sunday papers.

While some family members can rest easy in the cradle of family nurture, others may find the noise of children, and the need to fix the sink or walk the dogs, unbearable. The alternative of isolation and loneliness can be stressful: a time for those unhappy within themselves to live without the support of others.

Delegation and Resignation of Duty

It can be difficult to decline unwelcome requests: for another late night; an urgent meeting or another phone call, especially when duty is involved.

I remember being telephoned at 4 am., by a patient who complained she couldn't swallow! I wondered what she was trying to swallow, and why she had woken me to impart this vital news. Symptoms can provide key information which needs exploring, but not usually at 4 am! Next day I found her depressed. She was concerned about her son's imminent marriage to an unsuitable girlfriend (her opinion, not his). Her powerlessness was the root cause of her psychosomatic problems, not gullet cancer. Although those with early signs of cancer can deny symptoms, those with psychological symptoms are often keen to share them at 4a.m!

Sleep Induction

In the early days of commercial television, some adverts depicted a family before bedtime, peaceful and gathered around a fire, drinking a warm milky drink. The picture showed an ideal sleep induction process – a gradual, relaxed decline of arousal – rather than any sudden immersion. Watching a disturbing film, or engaging in arguments before sleep; trying to sleep in adverse physical conditions (light, heat, noise), or having drunk too many alcohol or caffeine loaded drinks, can all create agitation and make sleep induction difficult.

The same principle of premedication applies to anaesthetic practice. A patient brought frightened and screaming to an operating theatre, will need more anaesthetic to render them unconscious, than a relaxed patient. Effective pre-medication is thus important in the management of anaesthesia. Pre-operative awareness and alertness are best reduced.

Many people have a favourite sleep induction method. Some prefer to listen to music, read a book, or have sexual intercourse. Having fetishes that require a special time, place, and format for sleep induction are inadvisable.

Sleep Hygiene

Simple strategies can help with an inability to sleep: wearing eye patches for disturbing light conditions, and earplugs in a noisy environment. These can suffice for external annoyances, but equally disturbing are the stresses requiring mental processing, perhaps rehearsed during REM sleep.

The benefits of a comfortable bed and a pleasant place to sleep need not be challenged, although not all will care. Individuals might have a choice between a hammock, a waterbed, a king sized bed, or a beach with a rolled-up towel for a pillow. The preference for a certain ambient temperature can range from icy – windows fully open in winter (or with air-conditioning) – to tropical heat and high humidity. Those who are adaptable are more easily satisfied, but adaptability can suffer in association with TFE symptoms. Obsessive patients and those with TFE symptoms are easily annoyed by distractions. They may demand specific sleeping arrangements, and like Goldilocks, everything has to be 'just right' before considering sleep. Those with TFE symptoms are often irritable and easily annoyed. Although an irritable state denies them sleep and relaxation, not all will acknowledge it. This denial can make their clinical sleep management difficult.

Drugged Sleep

Taking sedatives is now deprecated by a medical profession, more concerned with addiction and accountability than TFE management. The risk of addiction is real, whereas the consequences of TFE symptoms are less often accounted for. Few TFE related topics appear in textbooks of medicine.

There can be little doubt about the efficacy of benzodiazepines in relieving anxiety and acquiring restful sleep. Anti-depressants do not quite match their efficacy, but are non-addictive. CBT works well but is time-consuming. All doctors want to avoid producing benzodiazepine addiction, but the effects of chronic sleep deprivation can carry a greater risk.

The prescription of all drugs needs personalisation. With benzodiazepine use, it is important to recognise addiction-prone and addiction resistant individuals. Typically, addiction resistant subjects dislike all medication, and are often anxious about side-effects. The addiction-prone worry less, and will readily embrace the experiment. Self-discipline varies between individuals and can relate to how readily they become addicted. The assumption that everyone will become addicted to sedative drugs is incorrect. For the moment, we must rely on clinical judgement of individual patients, and the balance of their likely risk and benefit, to make therapeutic decisions.

Many doctors concur: substance misuse, not the substance itself, is the issue.

Some sedative drugs, like benzodiazepines, are chemically harmless, as safe as the water that flows through the taps of London, UK. The adverse side-effects of liberally used alcohol and tobacco are significantly greater. Diazepam, in particular, sometimes uncovers depression. Despite its addictive nature, I have witnessed it freeing patients from chronic over-anxiety, enabling them to live normal lives. Although addictive, over many decades, I never encountered a toxic side-effect. Although people can use benzodiazepines for suicide, and the use of sedatives remains controversial, few will deny the value of relaxation, effective sleep induction, and restful sleep. These benefits (as referenced here) far outweigh any injudicious use of sedative drugs. This is especially so when they are prescribed by experienced and informed physicians who know their patients and are aware of abuse.

Withdrawal from an addictive drug given to promote sleep rarely presents a problem, especially when the most suitable patients are selected, and the timing of withdrawal is carefully chosen. Benzodiazepine withdrawal can be troublesome, and usually the only price paid by patients for taking them. Withdrawal is not as alarming as any heart attack or stroke, made more likely by disturbed sleep, in those at risk. I always allowed patients to withdraw while on holiday, when a few sleepless nights and anxious days, are tolerable. This is a small price to pay for years of improved, albeit not 'normal' sleep quality, and improved relaxation and composure throughout troublesome times. One important proviso pertains to the management of addictive sedatives: their success and safety is most easily achieved when taken by intelligent, compliant patients, who have concerns about addiction, with no wish to perpetuate it. Although their prevailing stress may not be soon removed, they will know that early withdrawal is to be encouraged.

One strategy for managing addictive drugs works. It is to prescribe three drugs to be used in rotation; alternating each one over two to three weeks. Intractable addiction to one drug will have less time to develop. This technique is especially useful for doctors dealing with high-risk patients, such as those with known severe ischaemic heart disease (deteriorating angina, recent cardiac infarction), resistant hypertension, or a recent transient TIA, where avoiding TFE symptoms might be of paramount importance. Doctors must then balance the risk of addiction with that of medical catastrophe.

It remains common for doctors to prescribe only ten tablets of diazepam to bereaved patients. This suggests that addiction (and regulation), are more concerning to them than the risk of TFE symptoms. We must compare the risk of bereavement to the risk of sedative drug addiction; however, several less addictive, though often less effective, alternatives to benzodiazepines exist. Consider also antihistamines, antidepressants, herbal medication (valerian) and CBT.

Once the problems causing TFE symptoms become resolved, quitting sedative drugs is usually easy. When the adaption process is likely to be prolonged, as with bereavement, psychological adjustment may take six to twelve months. Taking a safe drug for this period, combined with counselling, should allow for quicker adaptation. Unlike bereavement, some ongoing stresses will have finite solutions. After finding an acceptable solution, successful drug withdrawal may take only a few days.

Using data derived from a Medicare-based cohort of black and white married couples (aged 67 to 98 years at baseline; n = 373,189, in the US between 1993 and 2002), all-cause mortality increased by 18% (OR: 1.18) for men, and 16% for women (OR: 1.16), after the death of their spouse. A wife's death increased the risk of the spouse's death, by more than 20%. The major causes: chronic COPD, diabetes, accidents or serious fractures, infections or sepsis, cancer and all other known causes. The effect exceeds 10% for seven more causes of death: colon cancer, ischemic heart disease, congestive heart failure, nephritis, or kidney disease, cerebral vascular accident, or stroke, other heart and vascular diseases, and other cancers (Elwert, F., & Christakis, N.A. 2008).

The stress of bereavement in those of average age 55-years increased the likelihood of death by 40%, mostly in the second year after the death of their spouse. Not only the remaining spouse suffers. Many more close relatives (mean age 71 years) also die, in the four years following the death (seven times more than in control subjects). The subsequent death of relatives is highest when the death took place at a distant location. It was also more when the death occurred in hospital, rather than at home (Rees, W.D., Lutkins, S.G. 1967).

The Siesta

Afternoon napping is an important strategy for TFE symptom avoidance. Common misconceptions about short-term sleep exist. Many believe that an afternoon nap will reduce their ability to sleep at night. In fact, the relaxation that often ensues from napping allows for better night time sleep induction. Some think napping is a waste of time. I have heard said, 'I've paid a lot of money for this holiday. I will not waste it in bed!' They are perhaps more concerned about value for money than health.

Those who choose to treat TFE symptoms by taking a holiday may need five consecutive days of siesta, in order to experience a significant improvement. The holiday effect—the promise of pleasurable 'down-time' and reduced arousal, can make siestas attractive.

Chapter Seven

The Causes of TFE Symptoms

The following are assumed:

1. That cerebral activity (cognition, emoting and executive functioning) needs power for energy dependent neurophysiological processes.

2. The power used for cerebral activity depends on the time taken and the difficulty encountered (equivalents of volume and resistance).

3. The power spent on cerebral activity is modified by psychological factors: whether the activity brings joy and satisfaction or is tedious and unfulfilling. In the latter case, increased resistance to the activity spends more energy and will more likely cause TFE symptoms.

4. Tiredness as a presenting symptom can result from the underuse or overuse of cerebral power.

5. Fatigue and exhaustion are associated with the excessive use of cerebral power; less being achieved with unit power

used.

6. In normal subjects, increasing arousal 'A' (level of pressure, motivation, or stimulation) leads to increasing performance 'P', measured as work achieved in unit time (Fig. 1).

7. The gradient of the P v A relationship reduces as TFE symptoms extend from tiredness, through fatigue to exhaustion. (Fig 2).

8. With arousal near the tolerable maximum, performance will plateau or drop off in every TFE symptom state (Figs. 1 & 2).

9. With maximal stimulation, a sudden, bi-stable state can occur — a catastrophic drop in performance to zero, occurring after one small increment in stimulation. (Fig 2).

10. The normal energy (E) spent versus performance (P) relationship will be improved by athleticism and reduced in illness, recovery and exhaustion. (Fig. 4).

Important clinical TFE symptoms will occur in the absence of replenishing sleep (sleep deprivation). If prolonged enough, fatigue leading to exhaustion and medical catastrophe are possible (the sudden onset of failure to cope mentally, schizophrenia, depression, panic attacks, migraine, gout, worsening psoriasis and eczema, angina occurring with less effort, peptic ulceration, infection, resistant hypertension, stroke, or heart attack).

Although I have witnessed these scenarios as chronic TFE symptoms progress in severity, they frequently occur in patients with no obvious TFE. A pre-morbid disposition or the subclinical existence of these conditions is required before being exaggerated in association with TFE. TFE symptoms can also exist, with no associated clinical problems, usually the result of enduring, unresolved stress and defective sleep.

Significant problems face physicians. First, they need an interest in psycho-social matters, and may not see this as part of their job description. Second, they may not have time for the in-depth patient interrogation required (personal circumstances and stress factor evaluation).

I have discovered that evaluating TFE symptoms in complex cases helps explain why certain individuals become ill; why some remain ill, and why some deteriorate unexpectedly. Some made of sterner stuff will shrug off major stressing influences, either through indifference or through a constitutional, reduced liability to strain effects. Such differences are likely to be of evolutionary significance; survival favouring those who are resilient. Also, some will adapt more rapidly than others.

Most of us live with a sleep paradox, being unable to sleep well when stressed by unresolved problems. From an evolutionary perspective, the incitement of more REM sleep (perhaps for problem review), can reduce daytime energy and performance. This state reduces the likelihood of successful problem solving. In some circumstances, as in wartime or times of civil unrest, this could compromise survival through a failure to cope.

In exhaustion, where diminished performance follows increasing arousal, fear, anxiety, restlessness, and problem rumination will make sleep induction more difficult. The paradoxical sleep that occurs in response may be broken by periods of anxious wakefulness, nightmares and panic, accompanied by sweating and tachycardia. Even though some dreams are disturbing, they may need to be repeated. The result is unrefreshing sleep, daytime tiredness and a reduced ability to take action and solve problems.

Myalgic Encephalitis (ME)

As a form of 'Chronic Fatigue Syndrome', this is an ill-defined diagnostic entity, characterised by constant physical and mental tiredness for no obvious reason. The official US government website (cdc.gove/me-cfs/hcp/clinical) reports 3.3 million sufferers in the USA. The recognised features are fatigue not improved by rest (for more than six months), cognitive impairment, pre-exertional malaise and unrefreshing sleep.

Tests rarely reveal a specific viral cause, although in 80%, a post-viral illness is likely. The viruses detected include: EB virus, other herpes infections, parvovirus B19, Coxsackie B, enterovirus and borna disease virus (BDV) and SARS-CoV-2 (the cause of COVID-19). In a review of the scientific literature (Hyuang, J-H. 2023), found evidence for more viral infections in cases of ME/CFS (antibody and antigen detection), than in control subjects (ORs: 2–3.5 for BDV when comparing approx. 5000 ME/CFS subjects, with 9000 controls). Most frequently found were BDV, parvovirus B19, and Coxsackie B virus.

Apart from the possibility of a post-viral state, not every patient will have experienced inescapable stress or suffered depression, although the condition can itself be depressing. It occurs more in twins than expected, although no genetic predisposition has yet been found. It is not considered a psychological illness, though the thoroughness of each psychosocial enquiry needs questioning.

Orthostatic hypotension and vaso-vagal syncope are features in common with all causes of prolonged immobility. Whether a low BP is primary or secondary to prolonged inactivity in ME/CFS requires evaluation.

Not all patients experience a full recovery, but it is more likely, the younger the patient.

Menopause

The hormone changes associated with the menopause can induce TFE symptoms, with concurrent amenorrhoea and hot flushes, helping to define the diagnosis.

Chronic Ebstein-Barr Infection

(Glandular Fever or Infectious Mononucleosis)

This lacks substantial proof as a common cause (Hyuang, J-H. 2023). In my experience, many healthy subjects have had sub-clinical EB virus infections. I found raised EBV antibodies present in most CFS/ME cases, although I found only two out of fifty cases with constantly raised IgM antibodies, rather than the more usually raised IgG antibodies. Because I did not measure viral antigen, I was never sure whether the antibody changes represented recovery or an active infection phase. I gave some with raised antibodies, a two to three week course of doxycycline or oxytetracycline. Eighty percent of patients improved. Without being double-blinded, I could not be sure of a placebo effect, although most patients had tried various other medications without success.

These findings indicate the need for a double-blind trial. This is because:

- Although EBV is an DNA virus, all viruses must express their genes as functional mRNAs early in infection, in order to synthesise viral proteins (Rampersad, S. 2018). Since doxycycline and other tetracyclines can inhibit RNA replication, there is reason to support their use.

- Doxycycline binds to synthetic, double-stranded RNAs, and will inhibit their cleavage by RNase III. It could inhibit the normal processing of bacterial rRNA (Chukwudi, C.U. and Good, L. 2019).

- The binding of tetracyclines to double-stranded RNA helixes may alter the normal processing and functioning of the various biological processes they regulate. This could help to explain the wide range of action of tetracyclines acting against various pathogens and disease conditions. (Chukwudi, C.U., Good, L. 2016).

- Doxycycline and tetracyclines have multiple uses, one of which is to treat Dengue, COVID-19 and SARS-CoV-2 (Yates. P.A. et al. 2020).

- Minocycline (20 mg/kg) can attenuate IL-1β expression in the brain, reduce transient fever, and decrease spontaneous locomotor activity in rats (Kataoka et al., 2013).

There are many examples of CFS/ME following recovery from an illness, especially when post-viral.

Un-named Virus Infections

In everyday GP practice, the blaming of 'a virus' to explain why a patient is unwell or unduly tired is common practice. TFE symptoms are common before and during virus infections, including common upper respiratory tract infections, influenza, herpes simplex, herpes zoster, and many with viruses left unidentified. Even using guesswork, it is surprising how often the diagnosis will prove correct within one day or two. The problem is to differentiate trivial infections from more serious ones causing pneumonia, myocarditis, meningitis, and septicaemia.

Post-Traumatic Stress Disorder

The DSM-5 Diagnostic Criteria for PTSD details definitions for this diagnosis. 2014. (Exhibit 1.3-4).

PTSD results from adults experiencing a traumatic event and being exposed to the possibility of death, injury, or violence. Repeated exposure is likely to occur in those employed in policing and the armed forces.

The symptoms, which include those of TFE, include disturbed sleep with distressing dreams and daytime flashbacks. Other features are defective memory and feelings of negative self-worth with persistent anger, fear, and guilt. Reduced social involvement is a feature, with an inability to feel closeness, happiness, or satisfaction. Irritability, reckless behaviour, and startled responses are common. De-personalisation and de-realisation can occur with patients failing to engage with others.

TFE symptoms occur with disturbed sleep, combined with persistent daytime negative thoughts, fears, and concerns about current adequacy and future security.

Metabolic Causes of TFE

Blood glucose is the primary energy source for generating ATP in the brain, with glycogen as an important energy reserve, synthesised from glucose in astrocytes. Glycogenolysis and glycolysis reduce glycogen to lactate as a neuronal energy substrate in astrocytes transported by monocarboxylate transporters (MCTs).

Exhausted bees are quickly revived by giving them honey or a glucose solution or putting them on flowers so that they can feed on nectar (Quinlan, G. et al. 2023). In humans, TFE symptoms are not so easily reversed.

Brain glycogen decreases during memory tasks, sleep deprivation, and hypoglycaemia. Astrocytic glycogen-derived lactate is a critical energy source for meeting brain energy demands for neuronal functions and/or survival (Matsui, T. et al. 2017). They showed that exhausting exercise depleted both muscle and astrocyte glycogen. Failing endurance as a response to exhausting exercise has an astrocyte glycogen component. Is it possible that severe TFE symptoms are associated with astrocyte glycogen depletion, while glucose delivery maintains ATP synthesis?

Those debilitated by illness find physical activity challenging during recovery. They become easily exhausted, feel breathless, and have tachycardia after minimal performance. They will spend more energy than normal, achieving simple tasks (Fig. 4). Following such exercise, they may become mentally fatigued. Gaining physical fitness increases the ease of exercise, reducing any resistance felt, and promoting the feeling of reserve energy.

Fatigue in those over 70 years of age depends on co-morbidities and on daily physical activity. In one study, 77% of those over 70-years of age reported fatigue (van Seben, R. et al. 2019). Other studies support the correlation between physical activity and perceived fatigue ($r = -0.38$; $p < 0.38$)(Silva, J.P. et al. 2011), and total fatigue scores (Lin, W.Q. et al. 2015). Another study of older subjects found that active daily living was negatively correlated with fatigue ($r = -0.45$)(Karakurt, P., Ünsal, A. 2013). The relationship between physical activity and fatigue is bidirectional, with fatigue levels impacting physical performance. At all ages, therefore, the cerebral effects of exercise are beneficial. Perhaps fatigue in older subjects is exercise dependant, progressing as frailty and infirmity manifest.

Many diseases feature TFE symptoms, resulting from increased energy expenditure. More energy is required to maintain a body with an active disease than for a healthy one. Some of the highest risks as posed by CVS diseases (atherosclerosis and hypertension) and cancer, do not always present with TFE symptoms. Tiredness is not a feature of uncomplicated atherosclerosis and hypertension, yet both are potentially fatal. The same can be said for early cancers, despite their poor later prognosis. Chronic active infections like brucellosis, TB and those with abscess formation are notable for their TFE symptomatology. As differential diagnoses of ME, they are easily missed.

Sometimes tiredness results from toxic effects (alcohol, various drugs, heart failure, diabetes, renal failure, hypercapnia in respiratory failure and sleep apnoea).

Metabolic conditions can present with TFE symptoms. Thyroid hormone has many functions, most prominent of which involve the perception of heat and energy. Hypothyroid patients will feel cold in summer and lack energy; symptoms quickly reverse after taking thyroxine and/or tri-iodothyronine medication. Although much rarer, patients with Addison's disease can be profoundly tired, their energy being restored by cortisone medication. Diabetes can present with tiredness (diabetes fatigue syndrome; Kaira, S. 2018), and be associated with hyper- and hypo-glycaemia. Some with uncontrolled chronic diabetes are able to accommodate hyperglycaemia without fatigue.

The TFE symptoms associated with the menopause, can be profound and often reversed by hormone replacement therapy (oestrogen and progesterone preparations). Some women will gain daytime energy from taking androgen supplementation. Many younger women also suffer short-term TFE symptoms when pre-menstrual.

Chronic forms of anaemia, whatever the cause, are not always associated with tiredness. In my experience, it is more often associated with shortness of breath than tiredness. Untreated severe anaemia (Hb < 50% of normal range) can cause TFE symptoms at rest. Active GI bleeding that may cause anaemia, may itself be associated with unusual fatigue.

Physicians faced with a chronically fatigued patient have to meet an age-old diagnostic challenge. Is the cause psychological or physical? If physical, how are they to exclude every diagnosis?

How much investigation is appropriate? The patient might have to face a diagnostic grand-tour, being tested for every conceivable diagnosis, without a positive finding. If the patient has travelled to exotic locations, they may have an unusual infection. Advice from experts in transmissible diseases might be expedient. And so the search goes on!

From over one thousand cases that presented to me with TFE symptoms, as a component of their condition, only fifteen proved to have a definable diagnosis. Among them were leukaemia, myxoedema, Addison's disease, EB virus infection, chronic renal abscess, Weil's disease and Lyme disease. In all the others, ongoing stress, and disturbed sleep, were the commonest cause of TFE symptoms.

Cytokines and Neuroinflammation

Cytokines occurring with neuroinflammation are likely causes of fatigue, when a viral infection causes chronic fatigue. Their involvement in stress-related fatigue and depression etc., is less certain.

'Viral infections such as influenza cause the occurrence of acute inflammation, and pro-inflammatory cytokines including interleukin (IL)-1ß and/or antiviral cytokines including interferons (IFNs) are produced by activation of Toll-like receptors (TLRs) in the periphery.' Fatigue, depressive feeling, and cognitive impairment may occur concurrently (Yamato, M. & Kataoka, Y. 2015). A previous study with an animal model of viral infection showed these symptoms to be associated with neuro-inflammation (Yamato, M. et al. 2014). Neuro-inflammation is also present in Alzheimer's disease, Parkinson's disease, and depression (Song, C. et al., 2011).

It has also been shown that interferon alpha (IFN-α) in the brain modulates the serotonergic system by increasing serotonin

(5-HT) transporters, and can decrease running wheel activity in rats. These observations suggest that the production of IFN-α induces fatigue-like behaviour by suppression of the serotonergic system (Katafuchi et al., 2005). A COX-2 inhibitor prevented fever but did not improve their spontaneous running activity.

Peripherally-produced cytokines are thought to act on the central nervous system through multiple routes: (i) meningeal macrophages, cerebral endothelial cells, and perivascular microglial cells; (ii) cells which lack a functional blood-brain barrier; and (iii) vagal afferent nerves that innervate the nucleus of the solitary tract in the brain stem, projecting catecholaminergic fibres to the hypothalamus. Such afferent transductions of inflammatory signals are thought to induce activation (Yamato, M. & Kataoka, Y. (2015).

Electrolyte Imbalance

It is possible that electrolyte depletion and excess might cause TFE symptoms, but I only saw this rarely. Sodium and potassium loss can be associated with tiredness from dietary inadequacy, famine, or under conditions of extreme external heat.

Does the depletion of calcium, magnesium, manganese, selenium, etc. contribute to TFE symptoms, as claimed by many selling supplements? If so, their depletion would be a rare cause for TFE symptoms.

Dietary Influence

Vitamin B6 (from poultry, pork, some fish, oats, wheat germ) is a known co-factor in GABA neurotransmitter synthesis. Taken in excess, it can relieve anxiety and responses to stress (Duranni, D., Idress, R., et al. 2022). B6 deficiency is rare and associated with protein deficiency. It can cause tiredness and confusion in adults and seizures in infants. Its deficiency is most unlikely to be relevant in healthy adults with TFE in the western world.

Therapeutic Causes

Many drugs induce tiredness as a side effect. Some (like propranolol), can induce REM sleep and insomnia. Some drugs can cause patients to feel 'Tired All the Time'; among them are anti-histamines, tranquillisers and anti-depressant drugs. Most patients are aware of such adverse effects, and will stop them, or request their exchange.

CHAPTER EIGHT

The Personal Energy Equation

The brain synthesises high-energy compounds and spends energy on basic cell functioning, on neuronal activity, the conduction of depolarisation (neurotransmission), synaptic and cell voltage restoration. On a global scale, the brain spends energy integrating the pathways of depolarisation needed for each memory, cognitive processing, and emotional expression. As required by everyday life, cerebral functioning must respond to the environment and facilitate executive functioning. We can conceptualise the balance of energy creation and expenditure as a personal life equation, with standard format features and many individual variations.

The following assumptions have been made:

- The brain constantly creates and consumes energy metabolites.
- Sleep partly functions to restore daytime energy (occurring during slow-wave sleep).

- During sleep, most energy is spent while in REM sleep.

- Brain power is constantly dissipated at a basal rate (in a vegetative state, maintaining breathing and other autonomic functions), from unconsciousness and slow wave phases of sleep, to high activity alert states that involve active thinking (cognitive activity) and emotional responses.

- Mental energy dissipation increases with increasing cerebral activity (demands to think, calculate, and to process emotion).

- Tiredness is perceived at both low and high arousal states.

- The more mental work done, the more likely mental tiredness, fatigue or exhaustion (TFE) is likely to occur.

- Those managing stressful situations often suffer from insomnia (non-restorative, defective sleep), when restorative (SWS) sleep is what they need most.

- Continuing unresolved stress (weeks to months), with an unrelenting mental workload, can cause chronic TFE symptoms.

Some questions arise:

- Do TFE symptoms represent the depletion of high-energy compounds? or
- Neurotransmitter vesicles?
- Does it relate to cellular glycogen turnover/ storage?
- Do TFE symptoms result from blocked or inhibited neurotransmission?
- Does sleep release the daytime blockage of neurotransmission?
- Does the mental energy available 'E', equal what is stored 'St' (very small amount of ATP, but much more glycogen), plus the difference between energy synthesised (of ATP) 'S', and that used contemporaneously 'U', modified by plasticity 'p'?
- Therefore, can the flux of mental energy (E) at time (t), in a healthy adult can be described by:

$$dE/dt = St + dS/dt - p(dU/dt)?$$

- Is the total brain power (P) dissipated between two points in time, t1 and t2, proportional to the power (PVeeg) calculated function of the prevailing EEG, using voltage frequency (f), and voltage amplitude (A), with PVeeg = $2\pi fA$?

Namely, that:

$$\int P.dt\,(t1 - t2) \;\; \alpha \;\; \int PVeeg.dt\,(t1 - t2)$$

- If so, how does P relate to PVeeg? Can we assume a useful relationship, even if inaccurate, that might make the detection of TFE predictable?

Energy Homeostasis

If not mentally exhausted by sleep deprivation, physical toil can improve mental vitality and energy after exercise. Those already fatigued are easily exhausted. Digging up clumps of earth in a garden, filling wheelbarrows, and building compost can suffice to improve fitness. Perhaps the immediate beneficial effects relate to mental switch-off, while distracted from stress-related thought. Pumping iron, running on a treadmill in a gymnasium, running marathons and cycling up mountains, all have elements of the same benefit related to distraction. They can be contemplative activities with an element of meditation. Improved mental energy, with the brain re-set or re-charged during 'switch-off'. The perception of boosted mental energy also occurs with exhilaration, and endeavours successfully achieved.

Tiredness and sleep can result from situations that are boring and without motivation. This happens to those in prison, the retired, the elderly in nursing homes, and those relaxing on holiday. In these cases, tiredness does not result from high-energy spending, but from a state resembling hibernation. As with hibernation, normal functioning is restored only after some

Although those exhausted need re-charging sleep more than others, it may be beyond them if transfixed by constant striving (especially against resistance), or feeling depressed and demoralised. More often than not, the exhausted cannot take action, inactivated by mental inertia. Those who are fatigued could have energy enough to change their adverse circumstances. The disappointment of failure, however, will further consume any motive energy they have gained.

The strategy: WORK - WORK - WORK - COLLAPSE, is obviously less intelligent than WORK - REST - WORK - REST. Fatigued and exhausted people often lose clarity of thought, and may find it easier to continue with what they know (it saves some energy) rather than learning and adopting new skills (that require further mental energy).

The ability to 'switch off' and sleep, despite stress, has been a noted characteristic of few people. Historically, Napoleon, Florence Nightingale, Henry Kissinger, Ralph Nader, Winston Churchill, and Margaret Thatcher had been so able. This ability, especially if fostered by a noble cause, can act as a prophylactic for TFE symptoms.

It is possible to be replete with energy, having had enough rest and nourishing sleep during a holiday, only to arrive home to upsetting news; news bad enough to make one weak at the knees and unable to respond. Here, despite no TFE symptoms or fatigue, some experience energy blockage. A financial equivalent would be to have funds in a bank, but no means to access it. Both acute and chronic stress can cause mental inertia.

Having noble tasks, and being ruled by conscience, are not for every human being. In the film Chariots of Fire (1981), a steward wakes Mr Liddell on the overnight train from Scotland to London.

Steward: "Did you sleep well, Mr Liddell?".
Liddell: "Like a log".
Steward: "You must have a clear conscience then, Sir!"

Because it is so crucial to a worthwhile, pleasurable, and meaningful existence, many theories have developed about the function of sleep, some dating back millennia (Chapter 5). While the gods enjoy sweet sleep, and are 'happy in everlasting rest', we mere mortals become distressed through lack of it.

Distressed Penelope, the wife of Odysseus, became troubled by the fear of losing her son. Because of her inability to sleep, Homer offers advice. Written between 800 and 900 BCE, he writes:

'Sleep'st thou, distress'd Penelope? The Gods, happy in everlasting rest themselves. The Odyssey forbid thy sorrows. Thou shalt yet behold thy son again, who hath by no offence incurr'd at any time the wrath of heav'n. To whom, sweet-slumb'ring in the shadowy gate.' (Homer. The Odyssey. Book iv.)

What else has caused her insomnia? Homer gives her these words:

'From sorrows num'rous, and which, fretting, wear my heart continual; first, my spouse I lost with courage lion-like endow'd, a prince all-excellent, whose never-dying praise through Hellas and all Argos flew diffused; and now my only son, new to the toils and hazards of the sea, nor less untaught the arts of traffic, in a ship is gone far hence, for whose dear cause I sorrow more than for his Sire himself, and even shake with terror, lest he perish by their hands to whom he goes, or in the stormy deep; For num'rous are his foes, and all intent to slay him, ere he reach his home again.'

Homer. The Odyssey. Book iv..

One remarkable nurse proved far more perceptive than the doctors she worked with. She had been a child prodigy in European languages and mathematics. In 1854, when she led a group of nurses to the Crimea, Florence Nightingale, observed soldiers slow to recover from their wounds. If they had been fighting on the front line for an exhausting length of time, their wounds failed to heal. The wounds of soldiers freshly arrived healed fast. This observation, first made 170 years ago, has gradually accrued scientific support and understanding.

A meta-analysis of 300 published articles describing the relationship between psychological stress and immune parameters in humans found that acute stressors (lasting minutes) were potentially adaptive, upregulating some immune parameters and downregulating others. Brief stressors suppressed cellular immunity but preserved humoral immunity. Chronic stressors cause suppression of both cellular and humoral immune responses. The effects varied with the perception of trauma and any related loss (Segerstrom, S.C. & Miller, G.E. 2004).

Immune responses to stress are not limited to infection. For children, atopy increases after relocation abroad (Anderzen, I. et al.1997). Short-term stress can boost the immune system, but chronic stress may manifest as illness. Raised catecholamine and suppressor T cells levels can both suppress the immune system. This suppression increases the risk of viral infection (Salleh, M. R. 2008).

For decades, Florence Nightingale suffered debilitating fatigue herself, following her service in the Crimea. Once called Crimean Fever, brucellosis was the most likely cause. It did not diminish her achievements.

While she was serving in the Crimea, she reduced the mortality of hospitalised soldiers to under 2%, providing the statistics that persuaded military authorities to improve health care and nursing. By supplying the relevant statistics in a new form for the causes of mortality (as the first 'pie-chart' – the Coxcomb chart – which she invented), she influenced a Royal Commission's revision of the British Army's medical and purveyance systems. She revolutionised nursing training and established the Nightingale School of Nursing at St. Thomas' Hospital, London, in 1860. (Selanders, L. 2024).

Human energy expenditure at different scales (order of magnitude):

- At the molecular level (ATP and glycogen considerations);

- At an organ level (heart and brain functioning);
- At an 'internal', personal level: neuroticism, Type A & B behaviour; cognitive functioning / problem solving. Emotional functioning: coping with relationships and discord, while trying to achieve satisfaction, happiness, and ambitions.
- At an 'external', personal level: coping with everyday necessities: acquiring food, negotiating travel, climatic change adjustment, etc.
- At a societal, interactional level at work, and with family and friends. Cultural and political challenges.
- At an environmental level (housing, security; the supply and demand of utilities and products: facilities available, and travel possibilities. Responding to climatic and economic change.

The healthy interaction between each level will depend on timing, the order in which each presents, and their coordination. Getting food must precede the molecular use of nutrients. Poverty affects food supply, safety, security, and future risk. Poverty also affects ambition, hope for the future, and the ability to cope with everyday environmental conditions.

I do not consider diet here, but I acknowledge its importance to energy supply. Famine causes TFE symptoms, but this search for general causes of TFE in the Western world excludes it. Although life is impossible without adequate nutrition and its digestive processing, mental energy is many steps removed from considerations of dietary nutrients, fluid intake, electrolytes, fat, carbohydrate, protein, and vitamins. The focus here is where fully functioning sentient human beings spend, choose to spend, or need to spend their energy, and how they restore it.

Personal Energy Spending

One can classify the need to spend mental processing energy (in both the short and long term) as:

- Internal (resulting from neuroticism; Type A & B; cognitive and emotional functioning: dealing with challenges and problem solving, pain, insecurity, resentment, anger, fear, etc., or
- External (dealing with relationships, changing circumstances and living conditions. Dealing with discord; work issues, pursuing satisfaction, happiness, and ambitions).

In basic social terms, energy has to be spent getting food and shelter. Hunter-gatherers and their modern equivalents (those who live day to day with an unstructured life) spend most of their time engaged in related activity (as seen in nomadic tribes, and those detached from modern western civilisation). Individuals who have established a life through education or entrepreneurship, and now have a household and family, encounter maintenance challenges. Reversing the natural progression of diminishing entropy requires energy. The entropy principle is key, since energy has to be spent maintaining the status quo. Security and predictability need to be maintained by individuals, creating a safe path for themselves, their business, their home, and family. We also need energy for growth, perhaps to make additional high-entropy structures. With diminishing entropy, many will sense that their life is falling apart.

Other than at a personal level, external energy spending occurs at frontiers. Once urban citizens step beyond their front door, they must cope with pollution, traffic, noise, overcrowding, insecurity, political and social change. In the workplace, they must deal with financial and employment considerations, bounded by evermore rules, regulations, and regulators.

It is obvious from everyday experience that a spectrum exists between those who are physically and mentally active and those who are not. Ambitious individuals actively pursue their goals, while others passively exist, responding solely to compulsion. The internal drivers of behaviour derive from individual psychology: from ambition fuelled by ego and deprivation; love induced by caring and attraction, to dislike fuelled by discord and resentment. From neuroticism like obsession and anxiety; psychiatric conditions like mania and stupor, and active, time-urgent Type A behaviour, to more relaxed Type B behaviour. The accepted rules and regulations of our culture and belief system, together with our hopes and ambitions, will influence the mixture of traits and behaviours we adopt, all of which are described in every canon of world literature. Our available energy will help decide our achievements.

In disease, normal functioning can become disturbed. Disturbed by the energy drain of infection, mental illness, drug effects, pain and much more. Not only anxiety and fear cause insomnia, the delirium of septicaemia, the lack of oxygen, and excess carbon dioxide seen in some lung diseases are also causes. Add to this the effects of anaemia, diabetes, and various hormonal problems, all of which can fuel or detract from the energy patients perceive.

Counter to these behaviours run individual sleep characteristics: those who sleep well, regardless of their environment or any challenges in life, and those who are insomniac or have concerns about how to deal with their problems. How well we balance the two sides of our personal life equation, determine what energy we can bring to pursuing life. Unfortunately,

'When sorrows come, they come not as single spies. But in battalions.'

Claudius. Hamlet. Shakespeare.

Claudius alluded to 'the poison of deep grief', the energy for which can be overwhelming for some. Relationships often cause our deepest sorrows. When reality cannot meet our expectations, many spend energy coping with or adjusting to the resulting grief and discord. These concerns are most often played out during the fantasy of dreams, resulting in disturbing, less replenishing REM sleep. Unhappiness and fear, anxiety and worry all promote the downward energy trend. A perceived worsening situation, beyond one's ability to cope, can cause depression and TFE symptoms.

Abuse impacts many individuals, necessitating effective coping strategies. It comes in many forms; some obvious, some not. Among them are physical abuse (unexplained bruises and injuries); emotional abuse (being bullied, threatened, ridiculed, disrespected, and demeaned); neglect; sexual abuse, and financial and institutional abuse. Poverty, wealth, socioeconomic class, and educational attainment powerfully shape all human affairs.

Life Change Score and Energy Dissipation

How well individuals cope with stress depends on genetic profile and experience, and the stressors and anti-stressors in the environment (Theorell, T. 2022).

Life changes are a measure of external energy drain: the specific changes in circumstances that need to be coped with. The updated Holmes-Rahe Life Stress Inventory (Social Readjustment Rating Scale: SRRS)(Wallace, D. et al. 2023), provides a list of life changes, with scores that reflect their psychosocial impact. The highest life change scores are: death of a spouse, divorce, marital separation, detention in prison, and death of a close member of the family, major personal injury, or illness, marriage, being fired from work, marital reconciliation, and retirement. Among the lowest are: committing a minor offence, holidays, changes in eating and social habits, major changes in sleeping habits, taking out a loan, or a change in school or residency.

The SRRS can assess suicide risk (Blasco-Fontecilla, H, et al. 2012), and the likelihood of atopic dermatitis (Wardhana, M. et al. 2020). It has also been associated with the severity of coronary artery disease, although in one group, the results did not achieve statistical significance (Bagheri, B., et al. 2016). The SRRS inventory also failed to predict imminent myocardial infarction (MI) (de Faire, U.. Theorell, T. 1976). In another, longitudinal study, the life change score did not predict the occurrence of MI, but self-rated type A behaviour (high-energy expenditure) and dissatisfaction (long-term stress), predicted a significant number of near-future myocardial infarctions (Theorell, T., et al. 1975).

Acute stress, rather than the presence of long-term TFE symptoms, can cause cardiac infarction. Losing a significant person in life increases the occurrence of MI. In a study of 1985 subjects with MI, 13.6% had lost a significant person in their life, one to six months before; 19 occurred within one day of their loss. The calculated chance of MI was between 320:1 (for those at high risk) and 1,394:1, for those with no known risk (Mostofsky, E., et al. 2012). Whether the person who died suddenly had any previous long-term condition that had worried them, received no mention.

In keeping with the Whitehall studies, others have found an increased incidence of CHD in those who report long-term, adverse work conditions, low decision latitude, job strain or noise (Theorell, T., Jood, K., 2016). Others found long hours of work correlated with stroke, rather than IHD. (Kivimäki, M., et al. 2015). Perhaps TFE symptoms occurred in some.

Neurotic Traits and Energy Dissipation

Over long periods, those with fear, anxiety, and perfectionism traits are likely to spend more energy than those who are stoic and disinterested in perfection. A high prevalence of generalised anxiety disorder (GAD) was associated with chronic fatigue syndrome (CFS)(Fischler, B., et al. 1997). In a Dutch study of over 94,000 general-population subjects, CFS occurred in 1.3%. They were 1.63 to 2.32 times more likely to have anxiety than controls (Janssens, K.A., et al. (2015).

Sudden Death and TFE

Pain consumes energy. Many patients with chronic pain become tired as a result, but especially when their sleep becomes disturbed.

Coping with disabling conditions such as osteoarthritis of the hips and knees increases the effort needed for walking, and can induce physical and mental tiredness, sometimes leading to exhaustion. Patients will not improve if they cannot find enough energy for motivation. Under-stimulation and its associated tiredness can have morbid consequences; overstimulation and TFE symptoms can have fatal consequences.

Some soldiers in training, forced to march against their will, will get physically exhausted if goaded uncompromisingly. A few participants of public marathons, die as a result, usually within one mile of the finish line (0.8 per 100,000 participants)(Redelmeier, D.A. 2007). No pre-morbid indicators of sudden death among the runners were noted in this study. Whether any TFE symptom pertained is unknown.

In a retrospective study of sudden deaths (said to be 35 per 100,000 in the US), 41.1% had a prior cardiac symptom (dyspnoea in 17.8%, chest pain in 13.7%, palpitation in 1.4%, pre-syncope and syncope in 5.5%, and oedema in 17.8%), in the month before. (Keen, S., K. et al. 2021). In a similar study of sudden death, cardiac symptoms, but not TFE symptoms, were mentioned (Marijon, E. et al. 2016). TFE symptoms do, however, feature in psychologically-oriented studies. Apples and Orton found 'excess fatigue' to be the most prevalent precursor of sudden cardiac death, but only months before the event (Appels, A., Orton, F. 1992). The sudden death hazard ratio was 8.96 for those with exhaustion during the prior ten months. These patients reported: 'At the end of the day I am completely exhausted mentally and physically'.

The Health Divide

As sentient beings, humans have more in common than their differences, but it is our differences that attract more attention.

I have made the point elsewhere that wealth and poverty have different cultural aspects (The Art & Science of Medical Practice. Dighton. D.H. 2024). When immersed in either, distinct values, attitudes, and outlook form. The aspects that change most will depend on our educational background, our original family status and financial influences.

The reasons for the health divide have challenged medical science for decades. Why do the poor suffer more morbidity and mortality than the wealthy? What features of social class and ethnicity account for this? Whatever the social class, educational status, or ethnic origin, differences in morbidity and mortality are not just a few percentage points apart, but three to five-fold different. All developed countries show these disparities in cancer, cardiovascular disease, and infectious disease prevalence (Bambra, C. 2016).

The wealthy and the poor lead different socio-economic lives, in different locations, which can come to represent a different culture and ethos. Wealth and poverty affect lifestyle chances and attitudes, with differences at least as wide as those seen between distinct ethnic groups. The many differences between the lives of the advantaged and the deprived, must in part, explain some of the health divide. But which differences contribute most?

Smoking, alcohol consumption and obesity can account for at least 30% of the difference, but taken together, do not explain all the disease and mortality differences between the poor and wealthy.

A successful reduction in the industrial diseases once suffered by the poor (related to cotton, coal, and asbestos) has taken place over the last 100 years. There has also been a notable reduction in the number of people smoking tobacco (approximately 40% of people in the UK smoked in the 1960s. In 2020, only 13% smoked). Smoking cessation is an important feature of the health divide. Educated, high-earning individuals exhibit smoking cessation more frequently than less educated, low-income individuals.

To what extent do ethnicity and culture contribute to disease prevalence? In most countries, older adults, the poor, and the disadvantaged experience the highest prevalence of serious disease, while the rich and well-educated experience less. Disadvantaged groups experienced more serious consequences from COVID-19, with significant ethnic and cultural disparities in mortality rates. The BAME community in the UK suffered more from COVID-19 than others. The genetic basis of ethnicity, and the genetic material (RNA or DNA) composition of viruses, might have led us to anticipate some differences in how they interact.

The level of education we each have represents an important difference between us (Long, D. et al.2023); so does wealth and poverty, privilege, and deprivation ('Avoidable deaths accounted for 40.1% of all male deaths in the most deprived areas of England compared with 17.8% in the least deprived areas in 2020; for female deaths, it was 26.7% and 11.9%, respectively.' (Office for National Statistics [England]. Socioeconomic Inequalities in Avoidable Mortality. 2020).

There is a strong association between socio-economic grouping, disease prevalence, and clinical outcome. Cancer and cardiac infarction incidence are three to five times more common in deprived areas. Poverty is a major aetiological factor in the occurrence and prognosis of all the major causes of death in the western world. Could it be that coping with poverty requires more energy to be spent, and sleep that is more troubled? From a practicing doctor's point of view, both are probable.

Two centuries ago, the wealthy in first-world countries could afford to be obese, while the poor were undernourished and thin. The rich lived longer lives, and the poor shorter lives. To-day the rich in first-world countries have a lower BMI than the poor, and live longer. In poor countries the rich keep higher BMIs than the poor, yet live longer (Templin, T. et al. 2019). An important question thus arises. Which increases mortality most—obesity or poverty? The obvious scientific answer is poverty; the politically correct answer is obesity.

The Rich, the Poor, and Those Between

Compared to the rich, the poor more often have to cope with the stress of insecurity. They must work, or take social benefits, in order to get the bare necessities of life: food and shelter. If they want to maintain a higher standard of living, and encourage a better life-style for their families, they will have to work hard to overcome considerable expenses. This could challenge their cultural values.

The wealthy can choose whether they work, and need not waste their energy on insecurity. They are much more likely to be secure about their living conditions, unless their definition of security is to see their millions, or billions, grow further. Mostly, they can predict their future. They can choose whatever suits them, regardless of cost (rather than being restricted by limited funds and being controlled by others). The wealthy can have almost complete freedom of choice, regardless of cost. This comes together with freedom from any duty or obligation to others. This generates a distinct mindset and culture, unlike that of underprivileged groups. Many successful, self-made rich people often create their own stress. The poor have stress imposed upon them.

The middle classes ('the comfortable people of the middling sort', as Dickens referred to them) in the UK, represent a mixture of both cultures. Until they retire, and have paid off their mortgages, they will usually remain signed-up to many obligations. They do this in order to maintain their chosen lifestyle; to secure their future security and status, and that of their children. Their options exceed those of the impoverished, yet fall short of the wealthy. The middle classes desire status and recognition, which both the poor and the rich can abandon, albeit for different reasons. Middle-class stress comes from trying to achieve social homeostasis - maintaining the status quo. They strive to afford annual holidays, mortgage payments, school fees, car repayments, and taxes. They will do all they can to avoid poverty, hoping for a retirement without debt or work obligations. This demands high-energy consumption, likely to cause sleep disturbance.

At the moment, it is politically expedient (and fashionable) to blame food rather than poverty, for the three to five-fold morbidity and mortality found among the poor, when compared to the rich. Could the difference relate to the energy expenditure of constant toil, insecurity, and poor sleep? Naturally, many thrive despite poverty, and many wealthy people have a troubled life.

Humanity's challenges have changed over the last four centuries, with some reactions unchanged.

Art thou poor, yet hast thou golden slumbers?
O sweet content.
Art thou rich, yet is thy mind perplex'd?
O punishment.

'Sweet Content.'
Thomas Dekker (1575 – 1641).

How many poor people are content with their lot in life, and how many wealthy people care nothing about their bank balance and what they own?

If a lack of money leads to stress and discontent, why does dispensing money to the poor not always improve their quality of life? (Herrnstein & Murray, Free Press, 1994).

Marmot's findings (the Whitehall Studies), showed that ill-health and disease prevalence have much to do with the perceived control we have over our life circumstances (Bosma, H., et al. 1998). He compared the reduced morbidity of the executives in charge with those whose job is to obey orders. Naturally secure individuals experience less impact from stressful lives, perhaps because of genetic differences.

On one hand, we are told that our diet and growing obesity are claiming lives; on the other, we are all living longer on average, with less heart disease than during the 1960s. The rich can afford protein and will restrict their carbohydrate intake. They can more easily afford to be slim and fashionable. Not so the poor. Those who are poor and obese eat less protein and more carbohydrate.

Is it possible that obesity's impact differs based on socioeconomic status? Although mortality from obesity has important co-factors, like genetic profile, gut hormone production and affluence, personal energy considerations are not yet a métier considered by doctors or politicians, as a cause of the health divide.

Although the solution to poverty lies beyond the remit of the medical profession, health professionals have to deal with its consequences. The only politicians willing to address poverty are those resigned to retirement. No politician has yet convinced the rich to share their wealth with the poor; not unless a sizeable tax advantage accompanies it.

Neurotic Traits and Personality

There can be little doubt that neurotic traits like anxiety, phobia, obsession, hysteria, hypochondria and depression, can cause excessive energy expenditure. They are definite contributors to both TFE symptoms, sleep quality, and its recuperative effect.

Various attributes of personality affect sleep. The Five Factor Model of Personality (Digman, J.M. 1990), has five traits, based on William McDougall's five variables: intellect, character, temperament, disposition, and temper (McDougall. 1932). They are:

- Neuroticism. The tendency to experience distress and negative emotions;

- Extraversion. The tendency to experience positive emotions and to be sociable;
- Openness. The tendency to be curious and creative;
- Agreeableness. The tendency to be cooperative and altruistic; and
- Conscientiousness. The tendency to be self-disciplined and organised.

Extraversion and conscientiousness are associated with better quality sleep. Neuroticism, is associated with poor sleep (Stephan, Y. et al. 2017).

Time-urgent, impatient, rushing around, Type-A behaviour (Friedman & Rosenman, 1959), spends more daytime energy than its counterpart – Type B behaviour. The typical Type-A person is more aggressive, impatient, competitive and hostile. In a study of 764 older subjects in Wuhan, China, 44.76% were Type-A. The Type A group had a higher BMI, a higher proportion of CVS disease and diabetes, higher Hamilton Anxiety Scale scores, and poorer sleep quality (Zhou, X., et al. 2023). Their sleep was assessed using the Pittsburgh Sleep Quality Index (PSQI) (Buysse, D.J. et al. 1989).

Type A behaviour may be 'natural' to some, but can be induced (or revealed) in others, who experience time restricting conditions. Type 'B' characters typically make plans and behave in a leisurely fashion. They take their time and rarely hurry. They allow for redundancy in their time schedule, and plan for spare time.

Controversy exists over the contribution made by Type A behaviour to the aetiology of CVS disease. Interview technique is key for its proper evaluation, but many studies have relied only on questionnaires. One study showed that having Type A behaviour was an advantage, the relative CHD-associated mortality rate among Type A's was 0.58 (P = 0.03)(Ragland, D.R. and Brand, R.J. 1988). In a longitudinal study lasting 22-years by the same authors, Type A&B behaviour was not associated with coronary heart disease mortality (standardised relative hazard (SRH) = 0.9 8). (Ragland, D.R. & Brand, R.J.1988). In a more recent prospective study using self-reported scale, a relative risk for combined CHD death and nonfatal myocardial infarction (from controls) of 2.86 occurred for the highest quartile Type A scores (Kawachi, I. et al. 1998). Type A behaviour may act as a trigger for predicting when a CVS event will occur (Gallacher, J.E.J. et al. 2003). Because assessing Type A behaviour is complicated and unreliable, the QRISK3 algorithm excluded it as a predictor of CVS disease.

Status, Control and Energy Spending

The first Whitehall Study of British civil servants (Marmot, M.G., Bosma, H. et al 1997), demonstrated an inverse gradient between employment status and mortality: the lower the employment grade, the higher the mortality risk.

The Whitehall II study (Marmot, M.G. and Smith. G.D. 1997), found the following: 'that relative deprivation—a psychosocial concept—and the accumulation of socially-patterned exposures over the life course, must be important. Whitehall II suggests that the operation of these factors is to be found in the specific circumstances under which people grow, live and work.'

Eames, M. et al. (1993), found that: 'deprivation of an area and premature mortality are strongly linked. The effects of deprivation can be seen throughout the range of affluence and are not limited to the poorest areas.'

To arrive at this conclusion, they employed three different measures of social deprivation:

- The Carstairs Index (Carstairs V, Morris R. 1991).
- The Townsend Index (Townsend P, et al. 1988).
- The underprivileged area score (Jarman. B. 1983).

They noted the occurrence of various cancers, heart disease, cerebrovascular disease, respiratory and GI disease as causes of death. The highest weighted correlation coefficients between all causes of death, coronary disease and smoking-related diseases and deprivation (~ 0.5 - 0.76), were found in Merseyside and North East England. The least correlation was found in East Anglia (~ 0.17 – 0.34). Income and low employment were suggested factors. Smoking, diet and exercise are confounders, since those from the lower socio-economic groups smoke more and eat more fat and carbohydrate, while exercising less.

The first Whitehall study concluded that about 25% of the mortality gradient, could be explained by social differentials in smoking, plasma cholesterol, blood pressure, height, obesity, and physical activity. The Whitehall II study found that those occupations, characterised by a lack of control, were associated with increased CHD mortality; those characterised by high demand were not.

Low control was found associated with a raised fibrinogen levels (a measure of clotting tendency).

Not only job control appears important. People of lower status have different home and social conditions, and have experienced a different lifetime course, both educationally and socially. All of these could have contributed to their disease. It would seem, however, that low control is the most important of the factors (Marmot, M.G., et al. (1997).

The thesis developed here suggests that the occurrence of TFE symptoms is important for predicting the likelihood of morbidity and mortality. However, the Whitehall epidemiological studies did not include TFE symptoms. The current thesis suggests that, because of their job and environment, those at risk will be those suffering from most from TFE.

Environmental Energy Spending

Tolerance to road traffic and other noise pollution might develop best in those with no option to avoid it. Adaptation makes it bearable, but there will remain a constant subliminal stress, appreciated for its relevance only when it stops. Noisy communities are a source of stress and can induce significant increases in urine epinephrine and blood pressure (Seidman, M. D., Standring, R. T. 2010).

Making the change from living in a quiet rural location, to an inner city, can be a disturbing experience. For those living in the countryside, a distant owl might have woken them. In urban locations, many are engulfed in noise, much of which comes from the proximity of others: noisy neighbours, practising their singing and bonhomie at 3 a.m.

Urban dwellers who move to the countryside, may find it difficult to adjust to the silence. In any ranking of stress, this must be one of the lowest. Although the problem soon passes, it may leave rural dwellers sensitive to noise elsewhere – when travelling or staying in hotels, for instance.

One of the major considerations in comparing country to town living is the need for vigilance. A comparison of crime rates indicates that urban living is more dangerous than rural living. Crime rates for violence, sexual offences, robbery, burglary, vehicle offences, theft, and criminal damage are 50 – 80% less in rural areas than in urban areas of England (DEFRA. Crime. 2022). The need for vigilance is continuous, but an insensible, background stress.

Eames et al. 1993, found a greater correlation between mortality and deprivation in the densely populated areas like Merseyside and the North-East of England (densely populated), than in Norfolk (a rural county). Problems with privacy, living space, noise, overcrowding and pollution are more likely in urban areas. However, employment can present a problem for those living in rural areas.

In towns, residents frequently contend with crowds and round-the-clock activity that contrasts with rural settings. Town dwellers may prefer this to the relative quiet of the countryside. Swimming in syrup (urban living) will consume more energy overcoming resistance than swimming in water (rural living). Add to this, the vagaries of an overburdened transport system, and more energy spent on travel anxiety. Urban drivers will more often express anger, road rage, and other stress-induced behaviour. As traffic density increases, urban drivers will need more tolerance for increased journey times.

Much less personal planning and vigilance are required in the countryside, compared to negotiating the crowds of Oxford Street in London, 42nd Street in Manhattan, or Les Champs-Élysées in Paris. The need for small, impersonal transactions, like avoiding others on busy walkways, all consume energy. Urbanites need to be more alert than rural dwellers. The accumulative effect on health of many such minor transactions is unknown.

Town planning in the new towns of the UK has attempted to put space between people. Where space has been created, feelings of separation and loneliness can arise. The art of town planning is a balancing act. New towns and suburbia share the same predictable, boring quality; the economics of uniformity make it so, providing homes that are more affordable, and at the same time more profitable for construction companies. The retained identity and character of many old towns reduces traffic flow and increases human density, both inducing stress. There is an unfortunate danger to the boredom of uniformity: it can create the feeling of environmental imprisonment and dissatisfaction.

Many find rural life different, even boring. Cultural differences exist between nations. The French and the Russians prefer urban life (as reflected by property prices); many English people crave the peace of a rural cottage. British high-net-worth individuals frequently possess homes in both areas. They can reject the stress of urban living as and when desired. They can choose to walk through fields and forests, rather than crowded shopping centres. The low human density, fresh air, and the individuality of dwellings found in the countryside are special. Urban dwellers will remark, 'I don't know how you can stand living in the countryside, there is nothing going on!' A false, but reasonable impression. Socrates agreed: 'You see, I am fond of learning. Now the country places and the trees won't teach me anything, and the people in the city do (Plato. Phaedrus. 230d).

My family home was once near Saffron Walden, Essex, UK. Built in 1666, I am sure that no other house in the world is the same. While grandeur is unnecessary, personal taste can express individuality. Individuality, however, is restricted these days by building uniformity. Our ego drives us all to seek individuality, so living somewhere unique is one form of personalisation likely to generate self-esteem. The uniformity of flat and house design in towns can be de-personalising, with decreased chances for individual expression. One can only personalise them by choosing fixtures, fittings, and personal effects.

In UK villages, many residents know many others by their first name, although people don't always see social intimacy as an advantage. In towns, the inhabitants know few others, apart from their immediate neighbours. Valuing anonymity helps when choosing to live in an urban space.

For the health divide to reduce, perhaps modern socially-oriented town planning should allow the dispersion of towns into distinct self-styled hamlets, each big enough to support its own cricket or football team, with centralised shopping and other amenities. To promote health, spending less personal energy could be structured into the planning system.

Relative values are intrinsic to the understanding of human perception and judgement. What we are used to, and what we see as desirable, can underlie how we react to stress.

Surviving Relationships

By using discipline, heightened awareness, and a step by step analytical process to examine our mental processes, it is possible to resolve stressful, long held resentments and inappropriate responses to life events. The process would save energy, but few are inclined to pursue the challenge. The status quo may seem easier to maintain.

In my clinical experience, the commonest source of stress is inter-personal; either at home or in the workplace. Conflicts arise when there is a disparity between expectation and reality. Choosing partners based on attractiveness alone as the main discriminator risks incompatibility errors. Apart from dating agencies, using a psychological questionnaire would be unusual for assessing the suitability of a would-be partner. Procreation, not security or compatibility, remains the major evolutionary driving force.

In Oscar Wilde's The Importance of Being Ernest, Lady Bracknell (mother of Gwendolen), interrogates Jack to determine his eligibility as a possible son-in-law. She asks many detailed questions, but mainly about his education and financial status. In order to avoid future conflict in their relationship, she would have needed to compare their characters and primal needs.

The 'primal' relationship needs of individuals can be divided into three domains – affection, control and inclusion (Shultz, W. FIRO-B. 1950's). Discord arises when the affection sought by an individual is not received from a partner. Equally, if affection is not a primal need, discord will arise with anyone who offers it. The same applies to being controlled and being included in the affairs of others. Those who dislike being controlled, will be in conflict with anyone who tries to control them. The need to give and receive affection, control and inclusion, are basic inter-personal compatibility factors.

Perfectly matched needs are rare. If giving and receiving are the two attributes of three domains, the chance of a perfect match between to people is: 26 or = 64 : 1, assuming the three domain traits are evenly distributed among random candidates. This is unlikely to be the case.

If we assume that one in ten will reject affection, and one in ten will want to exert control over others, the odds of finding a match in a roomful of assorted strangers becomes: 64 x 10 x 10, i.e. 6400 : 1. In my experience, this is the more likely probability of finding a perfect relationship match.

Relationship problems consume a lot of cognitive energy; some requiring constant long-term expenditure. It follows that the majority of us will live with some stress from inter-personal conflict. Hence, the dictum: the ability to compromise is essential in every relationship (Gottman. J.)(Elmquest. J. 2017).

Surviving the Family

Family life can be supportive, edifying, or destructive. Babies and young children cry and need accommodating, while the feral nature of some teenagers often has to be tolerated, and perhaps disciplined by adults. Young adults have their own ideas, some of which will challenge long established family and religious culture. The first Whitehall study cited loss of control as a medical risk factor. Although this applied to the work environment, it could also apply at home.

Breast-feeding mothers must tolerate unstructured time. There may well be a mismatch of circadian rhythms between mother and child that can lead to exhaustion. Adherence to adult behavioural expectations can create conflict, made worse by poor sleep. Sleep deprivation can disturb composure and make mothers unable to cope. They may need to delegate their duties in order to sleep. Eastern cultures exhibit this more frequently than Western ones. Fewer western families offer the support found in third world countries. Many western mothers must learn to sleep when their child sleeps. Many become exhausted and feel out of control (Oakley, A. 1990)

Sleeping with children is one cause of cot death (sudden infant death syndrome). A parent might roll over in sleep, crushing and asphyxiating their child.

Whether by day or night, the distancing of a child from its mother can have unforeseen behavioural implications. Childless couples who can more easily afford a self-indulgent lifestyle might become shocked by parenthood. Single mothers with no family to rely on are liable to maximal stress and exhaustion.

Sleep deprivation will make any parental situation worse. To survive healthily (physically and mentally) as a parent, effective coping strategies need to be found. Mothers must learn how to cope with the relationship problems that arise. New fathers, side-lined by newborn needs, might seek comfort elsewhere. This will stress most relationships.

Pregnancy and child rearing have a strong evolutionary prerogative, and need an irrepressible biological drive to make them desirable. Having babies can be a trying and testing experience. Rearing children can consume large amounts of personal parental energy, not always accompanied by effective replenishing sleep. Parental changes in behaviour can result. Once parents have survived the early life of children, a supportive and worthwhile relationship can follow; something that improves longevity. A survey of those born in Sweden between 1911 and 1925, showed that couples with children lived longer than childless couples. Sixty-year-old men enjoyed a two-year life expectancy advantage; women, a 1.5 year advantage. The sex of the child did not affect the result (Modig, K. et al. 2017).

A Personal Journey

As far as human thought and feeling are concerned, the world has changed little since Plato, Marcus Aurelius, Shakespeare, or Dickens pondered it. Events such as bereavement, finding love, marriage, birth, death, and living through the agonies and ecstasies of relationships have remained unchanged.

In modern times, job security is an issue. Enough money is needed to pay for our chosen lifestyle. Any loans taken on, might necessitate paid employment for their repayment. Any insecurity will incite energy drain.

Those who pursue the equivalent of an opportunist, hunter-gatherer lifestyle will need perceptiveness, alertness, and intelligence if they are to be successful. Those with secure jobs and an unchanging lifestyle need less energy. These characteristics relate to social class and the health divide.

Applying intelligence, surveillance, objective analysis, and wise judgement are common traits among those who achieve their ambitions. With these advantages, they should be able to tackle life more efficiently – achieving objectives with less work – achieving more with less stress.

A recent phenomenon has emerged: the adaptation needed to cope with a fast changing world. The emotive message: 'you cannot afford to get left behind!', is seductive. New technology offers hope to those who are stuck in a rut and seek an escape. Faster travel and communication define modern life, but what benefits result? Contemplation and thoughtful thinking are more likely to give way to solutions. Some now seek avoidance of stress by viewing mobile phone apps. Social media platforms contain a mixture of correct information, disinformation, and inappropriate information that can all influence choice and behaviour.

Many get addicted to watching video reels and enticing adverts. The corporate profit motive thrives on dependency: trainers who offer the promise of wealth, if only we buy their training course. Usually, only the vendor gets rich. The prospect of easy money often appeals to those with little hope. On offer is they might escape the toil of making money and be able to boast about the new car or boat they own. Internet and digital marketing have created as many problems as they have solved, but good for business! The energy spent trying to escape our liabilities and energy spending can be defeating.

The conscious mind can be driven by many things: ambition, desire, doubt, guilt, and criticism, etc. During our formative years, we need to learn to protect ourselves by undertaking reconnaissance. This will help us avoid future pain. We doubt and distrust in order not to be hurt. Our negative 'mind talk' discussions can make life miserable, sometimes perpetuating misunderstanding and resentment. Sometimes mind-talk will be positive and elating. Most can keep their inner voices anchored to reality, but for some, constant analysis, criticism, suspicion, and doubt spend their energy.

Mind talk not only spends energy, it delays sleep induction, reduces slow-wave sleep, and heightens REM sleep. Many have followed Buddha, inspired to achieve nirvana, trying to achieve an uncluttered (low energy spending) mind. Few will emulate Voltaire's Professor Pangloss, whose assumption is that every situation leads to the best possible outcome; that this world is 'the best of all worlds' (Voltaire, F. 1757). Is it correct? Does an uncluttered state of mind always lie beneath the anger, pain, loss, depression, and abandonment of higher states of consciousness? Perhaps so, but this is only likely during slow-wave sleep, during anaesthesia, in a vegetative state, or near to death.

When faced with a conflict of conviction, dilemma can drain our energy. Resolving it can be life-shaping. Any search for an acceptable answer will not only pre-occupy the conscious mind, but may perturb REM sleep. The history of the British Royal family illustrates the stress of conflict between love and duty. The abdication of duty by Edward the Eighth for the love of Mrs Simpson; Princess Margaret's choice of duty over her love for Group Captain Peter Townsend, and Prince Charles, now King Charles III, who must have experienced the conflict of duty to his wife, the late Princess Diana, and his love for Camilla Parker-Bowles. A dilemma occurs when the future outcome of any choice is unpredictable. Princess Margaret could not marry a commoner and thereafter spent years in hedonistic displacement activity. Doing the opposite, Edward VII abdicated his royal duty for the love of Mrs Simpson. He afterwards spent considerable energy trying to regain family acceptance.

*One of my patients was suffering from chronic stress and had TFE symptoms. He was married, but in love with Sh****. His dilemma about what to do, trying to balance duty with love, had arrested a man used to decisiveness. When I asked him, 'can you see your future,* *without Sh**** in your life?', he shook my hand with vigour, and thanked me for the instant resolution of his dilemma. One question sharpened his resolve and removed his stress. It also relieved him of his TFE symptoms.*

Symptoms of TFE, caused by the stress of conflict, overlap those of depression. Common to both are irritability, defective memory, poor concentration, night waking, some sense of humour loss, defective decision making, and tiredness associated with defective sleep. Although we are all liable to TFE symptoms, only a few get depressed. I suspect this relates to an inherited pre-disposition, there being a greater incidence of anxiety, depression, and other neurotic traits among close relatives, than in a random cohort.

Chapter Nine

TFE Symptoms

Inflammation, Cardiovascular Disease, and Cancer

The inescapable duty of the exhausted British soldiers nursed by Florence Nightingale during the Crimean war, was to fight and risk death in conditions of extreme adversity (cold, heat, lack of sanitation, poor food, and drink). They lived with the fear of death, and no control over their fate. After injury and long deployment, they more readily succumbed to overwhelming infection. The same loss of control, important to clinical outcomes, was to become one conclusion of the Whitehall studies 140 years later (Marmot, M.G. et al. 1997). TFE symptoms result from many stressing factors (mentioned in the last chapter), together with defective sleep.

TFE symptoms are:

- Physiological (for tiredness and mild fatigue), a disturbance of the circadian cycle of tiredness – sleep – wakefulness, or
- Pathological (for exhaustion). Sleep deprivation, either

enforced or the consequence of ongoing fear, pain, and various forms of unrelieved distress.

Both can be acute (immediate cognitive and emotional processing), or chronic. Chronic TFE can be driven by several factors:

- Long term: slow, delayed cognitive, and emotional energy spending on unresolved or inescapable problems.
- Slow, background energy spending on what is not found exciting, motivated or positive, but draining, tiresome, boring, demoralising, inhibiting and negative.
- Negative feedback, from particular psychological responses once TFE symptoms arise: insecurity, fear, anger, frustration, resentment, and depression.

A lack of perceived available energy and poor motivation can lead to the perception of poor performance and further deterioration (a negative feedback loop). With a surfeit of perceived energy and effective performance, further improvements can result (positive feedback loop).

As TFE symptoms progress, from tiredness to exhaustion, decision making can become more challenging: misdirected, fragmented, uncertain and onerous. Clarity can be a challenge. Facing potential failure, some challenges feel insurmountable. The anger, irritability, and frustration that often accompany TFE symptoms will dissuade others from engaging with them. As exhaustion approaches, a catastrophic mental failure to cope can occur. Whether of acute or chronic origin, panic attacks, severe depression, or acute psychosis can render the subject incapable of normal executive functioning. In the physical realm, a heart attack or stroke, will represent a clinical catastrophe for the vulnerable—like those with significant hypertension [with left ventricular hypertrophy] or those with coronary or cerebral stenotic atherosclerosis.

Inflammatory Disease

Can TFE induce inflammatory disease? If chronic stress induces both pro-inflammatory factors and TFE symptoms, TFE might be associated with inflammatory processes. One review of inflammatory processes found stress linked to CVD, depression, neurodegenerative disease, and cancer (Liu, Y.Z., Wang, Y .X. 2017). One conclusion was that acute stressors can enhance immune function, and chronic stressors can be suppressive.

Several researchers have confirmed that stress can be pro-inflammatory, involving C-reactive protein, IL-6, TNFα, IL-1β and the transcription factor, nuclear kappa B (Miller, A.H. et al., 2009)(Elenkov, I.J. 2008).

Stress activates the hypothalamic axis and releases glucocorticoids from the adrenal cortex; glucocorticoids that are immunosuppressive and anti-inflammatory. Glucocorticoids reduce several pro-inflammatory cytokines (TNF-α, IL-6) and enhance some anti-inflammatory cytokines (IL-10, TNF-β)(Sorrells, S.F. et al., 2009).

Stress releases nor-epinephrine, and in rats, can release inflammatory factors within the innate central nervous, immune system (hippocampus)(Weber, M.D. 2015).

Inflammatory conditions consume energy. As well as the energy spent by inflammation, pain, and fever can cause disturbed sleep. High body temperature is associated with tiredness and an inability to move around. Rest is thereby enforced, although the quality of the rest achieved will vary with the severity of the condition. This is especially true in more severe conditions (malaria, pneumonia, sepsis), but less true for chronic fevers such as tuberculosis or glandular fever. Long, tranquil sleep is often a feature of recovery from debilitating illness.

A psycho-social challenge that evokes worry and leads to unaccustomed coping, increases EEG energy dissipation, and can lead to disturbed sleep. Without a sleep paradox, effective sleep would occur, regardless of stress.

In medical practice, it is common to observe a turning or breaking point, occurring in the natural history of an acute condition. Before antibiotics, doctors would await 'the crisis' of their infected patients: the point at which the patient's temperature abated and recovery was likely. This situation was sensitively depicted by Luke Fildes in his painting 'The Doctor' (1891)(Tate Gallery, London).

Over one century ago, doctors would assume that patients with night sweats suffered tuberculosis, until proven otherwise. I observed many patients with this symptom, each struggling with multiple stressing issues. Increased sympathetic nervous system activity during REM sleep can cause a racing pulse (appropriate for fight and flight) and sweating.

A turning point can also manifest as a panic attack, the onset of arterial clotting (perhaps causing a cerebral or cardiac infarction), or a bleed (perhaps a CVA). Other results are possible, depending on the physical and mental predisposition and status of the patient. Other events can occur like road traffic accidents because of defective concentration, repeated migraine, worsening psoriasis, pneumonia from defective immunity, or an illness that appears as if 'out of the blue'. In practice, these occurrences are the medical equivalent of physical bi-stable states, where one further stimulus can cause a sudden change (the snapping of elastic) – the proverbial 'straw that breaks the camel's back'.

The inconsequential nature of the final coup de gras, together with failing to recognise progressive TFE symptoms, can leave the timing of a medical catastrophe a mystery; the occurrence being assigned to serendipity (like other poorly understood phenomena).

Would-be preventative physicians need to recognise patients with TFE symptoms before any breaking point, and deflect their course towards recovery. The consequences of mental breakdown, heart attacks, and strokes are profound enough for them to be worth preventing.

It would be inappropriate to assume that TFE symptoms will always precede a medical catastrophe. The natural progression of coronary heart disease can take place without prior TFE symptoms. The more the genetic tendency towards atherogenesis, the greater the chance of coronary artery atheroma progression. Atherogenesis is slow, seen over decades, in some families (hence strong family histories of cardiac infarction). It is thus a pathophysiological process, likely to occur regardless of TFE symptoms. Whether TFE augments the process is unknown. Stress induced inflammatory and coagulability changes might, however, explain the association of TFE symptoms with sudden complete coronary artery occlusion as a catastrophe phenomenon.

TFE Symptoms and CVS Disease

Sleep and sleep disorders can affect cardiovascular function. Sleep disorders can affect the autonomic nervous system, cardiac rhythm and contractile functioning, endothelial function, and coagulation. Shift work, and sleep-disordered breathing with obesity, can influence the occurrence of hypertension, stroke, heart failure, cardiac arrhythmias, and sudden death (Wolk, R. et al. 2005).

Many reports have associated fatigue, sleep, and coronary artery disease. One study of 5419 Finnish adult men, found a higher prevalence of myocardial infarction in those who slept over nine hours, whilst more symptomatic coronary heart disease (CHD) occurred in those who slept less than six hours. The result persisted after correcting for many other factors, including Type A behaviour, medication, alcohol use, and hypertension. (Partinen, M., et al. 1982).

A meta-analysis of many published reports concluded that, 'Fatigue is the most common prodromal myocardial infarction symptom experienced by women.' (Blakeman, J.R., Stapleton, S.J. 2018). Most subjects were in their seventh decade of life. In a survey of male (n=384) and female (n=149) Norwegian patients (age < 75yrs), 62% self-reported fatigue in the year before acute myocardial infarction (also, dyspnoea 33%; chest pain in 45%). Fatigue as a prodromal symptom was almost three times more common in women than in men (Odds ratio = 2.97).(Løvlien, M. et al. 2009).

It has been long accepted that atherosclerosis is partly inflammatory, T-cells being activated by local antigens, presented by monocyte-driven macrophages that uptake lipids to form foam cells.

Macrophage activation leads to interferon-γ production, which helps regulate smooth muscle and endothelial functions. Raised IL-6 and CRP are both associated (Nadrowski, P. et al., 2016). Activated macrophages produce TNF-α and IL-1, which incite pro-coagulant, fibrinolytic and adhesive properties in endothelial cells. (Hanson, G.K. 2001).

In coronary artery disease, the degree of any arterial inflammation involved is an unlikely cause of TFE symptoms. It is only the occurrence of ischaemia, infarction, or heart failure that might be directly associated. It is more likely that prodromal tiredness, before acute myocardial infarction, results from stressing concerns associated with insomnia. In the research reported by Løvlien, M. et al. 2009, social circumstances, stressing problems, life changes and insomnia, were unreported.

Hypertension and insomnia are sometimes associated. Liu, D., Yu, C. et al. (2022), undertook a survey of the published evidence. Subgroup analysis showed that early morning wakening and insomnia were significantly associated with hypertension. They found a bidirectional relationship: hypertensives were more likely to suffer insomnia (OR: 1.2), and those with insomnia are more likely to be hypertensive (OR = 1.1). Poor sleep can also be associated with a need for increased antihypertensive medication (Hernandez-Aceituno A., et al. 2019). Treating insomnia and improving sleep habits can be important to the control other chronic diseases, like diabetes (Koopman, A. D., et al. 2020).

The slow deterioration of health that can accompany TFE symptoms can be a feature of pre-cardiac infarction syndrome. Having observed this frequently, I came to regard it as an important clinical screening observation. Acute infarction can occur without a prodrome, although verification from interviewing family, friends, and workmates is not always possible. The denial of TFE symptoms by patients is common, being thought by some, to indicate weakness.

Most patients with angina have mechanical, flow-limiting coronary artery stenoses, and the assessment and management of these must take priority over TFE considerations. Once intervention has reduced any ischaemia, longer-term TFE management might be considered next. If no cardiac intervention is possible (angioplasty or CABG), TFE management should take priority.

TFE and Cancer

Chronic stress can vary cancer outcomes (Krizanova, O. et al., 2016). It may also be associated with tumour aetiology, progress, and metastasis (Thaker, H. et al., 2006). In a three-year post-treatment study of breast cancer cases, elevated acute phase proteins were associated with increased morbidity and mortality (Pierce, B.L. et al., 2009).

Doctors typically classify TFE symptoms as non-specific in disease diagnosis. However, they result from active energy spending and sleep disturbance. They can indicate enhanced inflammatory processes and unresolved psychosocial issues. In neoplastic disease, TFE symptoms will not usually be present until the advanced stages of metastasis, with vital processes succumbing to insufficient energy.

CHAPTER TEN

The Clinical Management of TFE

Of grief and anger, a most potent charm for ills of ev'ry name.

The Odyssey. Homer. Book iv.

Consider some common clinical observations I made over many decades in cardiac practice:

- Many patients with innocent forms of palpitation (usually atrial and ventricular ectopic beats), vasomotor syncope, resistant hypertension, and refractory angina, sometimes had associated TFE symptoms.

- With TFE symptom reduction (from stress reduction or removal, and improved sleep), improved symptoms and management occurred many times.

- The resolution of stressful situations and improved sleep, required a psychosocial analysis of each patient's personal circumstances, followed by targeted counselling to make changes that aided adaptation. Not all patients could comply.

- The complete process took a variable amount of time, from immediate to many months.

- Removing TFE symptoms often improved symptoms such as palpitations and syncope, or reduced the need for medication to manage hypertension or angina.

From the above anecdotal observations, one could deduce that circumstances leading to TFE symptoms are important contributors to the frequency and/or severity of some CVS symptoms.

The beneficial effects observed are likely to follow improved pathophysiology. Reduction of sympathetic drive in palpitation, hypertension, and angina, and altered vasovagal influence, allowing vaso-motor syncope reduction, are plausible explanations. Improvements in pathological processes (atherogenesis, arteriosclerosis) cannot be claimed. Also, one cannot claim reduced risk of cardiac infarction or stroke in specific cases, although there is some evidence in support (see previous chapters).

Many doctors will prescribe a beta-blocker when palpitations might have an increased sympathetic autonomic component. Vasomotor syncope suggests an increase in parasympathetic activity. Beta-blockade can help, although propranolol can cause sleep disturbance. Although beta-blockade can work well in the short-term, better long-term management must involve the removal of instigating stressors. Combining both might be advisable. Many of my patients refused a beta blocker, so I could observe the direct effect of stress reduction, and improved sleep, on their symptoms.

Improvement of angina with improved TFE symptoms is less common. I did, however, observe a few cases where a sudden beneficial change in circumstances resulted in improved effort tolerance.

One case, which I mentioned elsewhere, was that of a fifty-year old man with angina and three-vessel coronary disease. He was suffering depression from bereavement, and had limited exercise tolerance. After finding a new, fulfilling relationship, his exercise performance improved without a coronary intervention or a change in his medication.

Since such anecdotal observations are common, further studies might prove worthwhile.

TFE Symptom Management

Since no neurophysiological equivalent of a battery exists in the central nervous system, the concept of brain 'recharging' during sleep must be incorrect. One might, however, apply the concept to the restoration of individual synapses and axons after depolarisation. Together with the dis-inhibition of synapses, 'resetting' is perhaps the best description.

TFE symptoms occur with continued cerebral energy spending, combined with the inadequate resetting of neurophysiological synaptic processes during sleep. It follows that to manage TFE symptoms effectively, three objectives must be achieved:

- To remove or adjust precipitating features (adverse life circumstances).To reduce the psychological responses to circumstances (anxiety, fear and depression).

- To reduce the psychological responses to circumstances (anxiety, fear, and depression
- The judicious use of psychotropic drugs when needed.
- To implement measures which improve slow-wave sleep.
- To introduce lifestyle adjustments which foster relaxation and mental detachment from causative situations (exercise, meditation, massage, holidays, distracting pursuits, hobbies, yoga, CBTi, prayer, etc.

Non-Sleep, Neurophysiological Re-Setting

Can we reduce TFE symptoms while subjects are conscious, or only during NREM sleep?

Several practices claim to switch off conscious 'mind talk' (thinking of nothing), and thus reduce energy expenditure. Among them are hypnosis, meditation, yoga, prayer, and Qigong (an ancient Chinese healing practice: meditation with controlled breathing and movement). All aid relaxation.

Yoga is a collective term for different practices. It has a modest clinical effect on lowering blood pressure (less medication needed). The three most important components are different postures, breathing practices, and meditation (Joshi A.M. et al. 2024). In a review of published work on yoga and blood pressure (Tyagi, A. et al. 2014) found the range of blood pressure reduction limited to 3–15 mms. Hg systolic, and less for the diastolic pressure. The long-term sustainability of this modest advantage is another matter. At least one can conclude that yoga can reduce blood pressure for some patients experiencing stress (with increased energy expenditure).

When the brain is 'switched off', but awake, it can produce EEG alpha waves (□ 7-13 cycles/second). Some believe that time spent in an alpha-wave state can improve attention and academic learning, but others dispute the results (Kim, S.C. et al. 2014). This state accompanies mental quiet with the eyes closed. Alpha rhythm can accompany hypnosis, yoga, and meditation, and perhaps represents neurophysiological resetting during wakefulness. During theta wave, NREM sleep, recovery from TFE symptoms may be more effective.

For centuries, a tranquil state has been associated by some with 'samadhi', 'pure awareness,' or 'enlightenment'. This state of consciousness has long been the point of Vedic, Buddhist, and Taoist practices. Transcendental meditation (TM) is a later, western addition. The physiological changes that can occur during meditation are: increased cardiac output, increased cerebral blood flow, cessation of CO2 generation in muscle, fivefold elevation of plasma arginine vasopressin (ADH or AVP), and EEG synchrony (Jevning, R., Wallace, R.K. et al. 1992).

In parallel with general anaesthesia, meditation can lead to various depths of consciousness (Katyal, S., & Goldin, P. (2021). Theta (4–6 Hz) and alpha (7–13 Hz) EEG oscillations relate to the depth of meditation, and the inverse of one another in frontal brain areas. Executive processing, monitoring, and attention are downregulated during deeper meditation experiences.

Others have compared 'thinking of nothing' to 'Qigong', using multichannel EEGs and sLORETA functional EEG tomography. EEG alpha-2 frequency in the right hemisphere differed significantly in 125 voxels; all were more active during 'Qigong' than

'Thinking of Nothing'. In the left hemisphere, beta-1 frequencies were more active in the 'Thinking of Nothing', than in 'Qigong' periods. (Faber, P.L., et al. 2012).

Because brain energy output reduction is important in the management of TFE symptoms, it is not surprising that meditation improves executive functioning and mental health (Leyland, A. et al. 2019). Autonomic activity changes, found with both meditation and yoga, can benefit the management of hypertension (Jevning, R., et al. 1992)(Hagins, M., et al. (2013).

The EEG changes occurring with TM and hypnosis are unpredictable, and not always repeatable. A group of meditating subjects showed significantly more theta activity (during both TM and non-meditation) than a randomly selected control group (Tebecis, A.K. 1975).

The five principles of yoga are:

- Relaxation: letting go of worries and fears; releasing tension in the muscles, and resting.
- Exercise: yoga positions, stretching and toning all muscles and ligaments.
- Breathing: rhythmic breathing exercises to control mental state.
- Diet: balanced and nourishing.
- Positive thinking and meditation: to remove negative thoughts, to still the mind and transcend all thought.

Some who practice yoga attempt to achieve a 'higher state of consciousness', expressed as the degree to which they can detach themselves from reality. Some gain a state of greater composure.

One can easily challenge the unscientific rationale behind many alternative beliefs regarding alternative therapies, but the reality of their benefits is not so easily refuted. Explanations given for why and how they work are often ill-conceived in scientific terms (lacking objectivity, being un-verifiable, and un-reproducible). Unlike scientific explanations, delusional explanations will mostly lack supporting evidence.

The accessibility of scientific information can bar public understanding. Scientific knowledge is hierarchical and based on established principles. Those without such knowledge are vulnerable to myths created using ill-definable terms. They may present these beliefs as stemming from a separate system of thought, inaccessible to non-believers.

An obsessional attitude promotes energy spending, and sleep that may depend on optimal conditions. Obsessive characters may harbour beliefs like: 'I can only sleep when it's quiet, and only when it's completely dark!' – 'Only with my special pillow!' or, 'Only with the windows open!'

Anything that reduces energy output can help to improve the perception of having energy. Prayer has a satisfying and recharging effect for worshippers of all religions. Conforming with a strict code of discipline, such as daily fasting, will not only raise the sense of personal dignity and integrity but also energise self-worth. Ramadan, Yom Kippur, attending midnight Mass, and reciting mantras are examples.

Based on personal circadian rhythm, there should be optimal times for meditation and relaxation. For contemplative meditation, a waking state is best. When trying to achieve a prominent alpha rhythm, choosing a low point in arousal might prove best.

A calm mind fosters purpose and decisiveness. Without the perception of sufficient personal energy, composure can be difficult to gain. Instead, many revert to busying themselves with daily duties, or acting out the dramas of life, with little resourcefulness to spare. In this aroused state, one can only deal with life as it comes. Planning for later events may be side-lined, and the future left to serendipity.

A lack of control may commit us to larger amounts of energy expenditure in the future. We may need extra energy to overcome accumulated problems—dealing with increased entropy—just to 'get back on track', or to 'put things back to normal'. The same consequences await those who, ruled by their emotions, decide on impulse rather than after intelligent consideration. Some consider that true living means going wherever life leads (analysis and judgement being suspended).

Sleep Management

During daytime activity, human executive functioning efficiency usually depends on the length and nature of the previous sleep period, although dependency on this varies. Some anticipate their need for sleep and plan it: choosing an early bedtime, and avoiding prior alcohol and disturbing stimulation (intense conversation or watching a horror movie). A quiet preliminary phase aids sleep induction. An untroubled mind will usually promote refreshing sleep. Correct sleep hygiene helps; sleep being promoted by reducing ambient noise and light, a comfortable bed, and suitable pillows.

Insomnia affects the disadvantaged, and some cultural subgroups more than others (Chen, X. et al. 2015). Sleep disturbance has a social dimension. The poor more often have variable work schedules and sleep patterns than the wealthy. For the poor, insomnia can be inescapable.

Sleep Therapy

An ancient Greek suggestion was that wine could induce desirable 'sweet' sleep (γλύκυς: glykis) for those like Penelope, stressed by Odysseus' absence (Homer. The Oddysey). The ideal was to sleep like Zeus' (described as γλύκυς), or like Agamemnon, described as ἀμβρόσιος ('ambrosial').

In 1942, psychiatrist William Sargent treated exhausted soldiers returning from Dunkirk to England during the second world war. He prescribed three-weeks of drugged sleep therapy, using amylobarbitone. In his memoir (The Unquiet Mind, 1967), he recounts using it 'for restoring the shattered nervous system of war casualties'. Before that, Emelio Mira y López had used sleep therapy for soldiers fighting in the Spanish Civil War (1936-1939)(Mira y López, E. 1943).

At Charing Cross Hospital, working with Dr. Peter Nixon in the 1970s, I was involved with short-term sleep therapy. We designed it to last three to seven days for patients with TFE symptoms and cardiac problems. Patients with IHD and uncontrolled hypertension were sedated if they had fatigue or exhaustion (with diazepam and promethazine). The aim was to make patients sleep over six hours every night, with two to three hours every morning, and the same after lunch. Patients were mobilised between each sleep period, and thus avoided chest infection, muscle and joint stiffness, and DVT. Few complications resulted. Achieving low-risk sleep therapy, however, requires specific staff training.

After two or three days of sedation, the patient's restlessness would disappear; they awoke less often, and their breathing pattern became more regular. They were perhaps spending less time in REM sleep, and more time in restful, slow-wave sleep. A slow pulse, quiet breathing, and low blood pressure were then characteristic. Parallel observations are appropriate for safe anaesthesia; the rate and regularity of breathing indicate the depth of anaesthesia. In deep anaesthesia, one can observe the same slow, regular breathing as in normal NREM sleep. Some anaesthetists now use EEG spectral analysis to confirm this.

Early on during sleep therapy, one may observe some physical activity during REM sleep. Sleeping dogs exhibit the same. Their movements, while asleep, might reflect galloping over fields and chasing rabbits while dreaming. Who can know?

Once recovered, we interviewed all patients. The aim was to discover the psychosocial reasons for their demise. With the involvement of their family, friends and work colleagues, we attempted to find solutions to their problems. Some required handling by psychotherapists and family therapists (now CBT-I specialists). Sometimes, one simple suggestion would solve what seemed to be a complicated problem. Here is one clinical example:

I admitted a 62-year-old woman with resistant hypertension. With her husband, she managed a small, family-run manufacturing company. She claimed her role required six days of work each week. She thought her role essential; without her presence, the company might not survive.

A different picture emerged from her husband, who founded the company twenty years before. When I discussed her essential status with him, he looked surprised. He said they had plenty of staff who could fulfil her role. He thought of her role as interfering, rather than essential. She had, in fact, refused to retire many times, despite her increasing tiredness, fatigue, irritability, and resistant hypertension. Pride and her need for self-esteem had made her continue.

The solution I suggested was that she should retire on medical grounds. This would preserve her dignity and reduce the risk of her having a stroke, given her resistant hypertension (something suffered by her mother). She agreed, and retired with her self-esteem intact. In follow-up, her hypertension became much easier to manage on less medication.

Not all cases are simple to resolve, especially when many parties are involved, and the patient regards their situation as inescapable. For the patient, a lack of insight, ignorance, and arrogance can block healthy change. Dr. Peter Nixon admitted that some were recalcitrant recidivists.

Tactical Napping

A NASA study (1995), found that pilots who napped for 26 minutes experienced a 54% increase in average alertness, and a 34% increase in performance, compared to those who did not. Those who napped experienced less sleepiness toward the end of their flights. The pilots who did not, experienced twice as much daytime sleepiness (Rosekind, M. R., et al. 1995).

More recent studies have shown other benefits (Dutheil, F., et al. 2021):

- Improved memory.
- Improved creativity.
- Decreased reaction time.
- Improved focus and concentration.
- Lower blood pressure.

Cognitive Behavioural Therapy (CBT)

The primary focus of CBT (or CBT-I for insomnia) is to address the factors contributing to chronic insomnia. (Walker, J., et al. 2023).

These factors include predisposition, like high emotional reactivity; precipitating factors, like stressful life events; perpetuating factors, like living and work conditions, including fears about the future, security, and relationships (Spielman, A.J. 1986).

Treatment usually takes five or six sessions. Each session has a specific agenda, like evaluation, treatment rationale, intervention, adherence, and relapse considerations. The objective is to enhance homeostatic sleep drive.

A key component (sleep restriction), will restrict any extended time in bed as compensation for poor sleep. By prescribing a sleep schedule, it can reduce the time spent in sleep induction, and the time spent awake at night.

Stimulus control therapy aims to remove those stimuli from the sleep environment that disturb induction: TV, books, radio, and social media. It directs subjects to go to bed only when sleepy, and to get up if lying awake for over 15-20 minutes. It involves daily consistent wake-up times with no naps.

Cognitive therapy attempts to create realistic expectations of sleep, and to dispel any misguided thoughts that might prevent it. Any maladaptive thoughts and reactions are examined and replaced with realistic thoughts, explanations, and expectations. The process is one of guided discovery. Sleep hygiene and exercise are promoted; alcohol and stimulant use, including caffeine, are discouraged.

CBT can reduce insomnia related symptoms by 50% to 80% (Morin, C.M. 1994)(Morin, C.M. 2009), with benefits that appear stable. Consistent improvements in daytime functioning are less certain. Because CBTi is at least as effective as pharmacological interventions, it is now recommended as the first-line treatment for insomnia (American College of Physicians).

Hypnosis

A review of twenty-four studies found that 58.3% who reported improved sleep after hypnosis; 12.5% yielded mixed results, and 29.2% reported no benefit (Chamine, I. et al. 2018). The study did not select patients sensitive to hypnosis.

Hypnosis treatment has the advantage of needing only a few short sessions. Adverse effects occur infrequently. It can also be used as an adjunct to other forms of psychotherapy. The place of self-hypnosis needs exploration (Elkins, G, et al. 2013).

Compared to Zolpidem, 10mgs for 14 nights, hypnotherapy can work well for those with PTSD, as measured by the Post-traumatic Disorder Scale. The benefits lasted for at least one month (Abromowitz, E.G. et al. 2010).

Distraction and Relaxation

Distractions are often used to aid relaxation; a daytime switch-off for productive people. Sometimes distraction is displacement activity, shielding stressed people from challenging situations. Listening to the twittering inanities broadcast on radio and television might engage us, but distract us from problem solving. Sometimes distraction is a parallel activity. Driving, for instance, allows us time to think and to solve problems. Repetitive exercise requires very little thought, and can allow new ideas and solutions to arise.

Personal success and acknowledgement often result in a feeling of exhilaration, with boosted self-esteem, happiness with contentment; a feeling of fulfilment with satisfaction. Such responses are progenitors of relaxation, effective sleep, and an improvement in perceived energy. Those needing resources frequently receive the least. It applies to wealth and energy alike.

Besides the physical benefits of training, are other mental benefits: increased confidence, improved sleep, libido, and vitality. Physical training enables improved attention, concentration, and focus. Those who train regularly, often accept these advantages as the norm. Fitness can produce a euphoric mental state, similar to that caused by some drugs: an experience that fosters further activity and a desire for greater fitness.

Whereas an unfit person might choose to relax or sleep, a trained athlete might choose to exercise. Active families are likely to beget physically active children. I suspect the inclination to be active or lazy is an inherited characteristic.

The Yekuana tribe, who live in the Venezuelan rain forest, view wakefulness and sleep as equally valuable. Often, all will wake at night to share a joke, or to observe a nearby wild-boar pack. They would then return to sleep, with no annoyance incurred. Jean Liedlof, in her book The Continuum Concept (1975), describes how the Yekuana respect both the inherently lazy (as viewed by western eyes) and the active, as having innate characteristics.

Relevant Clinical Diagnoses

Physicians have a duty to explore the physical causes of TFE symptoms. Among them, will be endocrine dysfunction: hypothyroidism, the menopause, and reduced cortisol availability. Diabetes is commoner, but only causes TFE symptoms when uncontrolled. Advanced inflammatory conditions can cause TFE symptoms, whether involving infection of autoimmunity. Apart from illness itself, being a patient requires effort; the need to attend clinics and to undergo treatment, can be fatiguing. When combined with worries about diagnosis and prognosis, sleep disturbance and TFE symptoms become more likely.

Because finding a discreet cause for TFE symptoms is unusual, several clinical entities might explain the mystery. Myalgic encephalomyelitis (ME), is one such diagnosis that has received WHO recognition. It has been used to explain one cause of chronic fatigue syndrome, with little evidence to confirm it as a clinical entity with specific enough criteria for reliable diagnosis. Is it psychosomatic or true brain disease? Various explanations are: traumatic life events, exhaustion of nervous system energy or neurasthenia (Beard, G. 1898), a neuro-immune disease, psychosomatic, a viral illness, mass hysteria, 'Yuppie Flu', or a biosocial syndrome, maintained by illness beliefs. The World Health Organization (WHO) has classified ME as a neurological disorder (International Classification of Diseases. ICD-10: G 93.3; WHO, 1992)(ME Society. Nursing in Practice: June, 2016).

Some patients with ME have raised inflammatory markers, autonomic imbalance (orthostatic hypotension), with occasional brain changes found on MRI scanning (Shan, Z.Y. 2020). MRI scanning has sometimes detected brain-stem changes in volume and myelination. These can be associated with clinical features, including sleep parameters (Nelson, T. et al. 2021). Whether these volume changes are the same as those seen in anxiety and obsessional-compulsive disorder (OCD), and PTSD, found in the hippocampus, amygdala, cingulate, prefrontal and parietal cortex (Bremner, J.D. (2004), has to be decided. Changes in myelination still need explanation.

Many have suggested that ME is not 'physical', but a psychosomatic condition needing psychotherapy. A review of the all-cause mortality of ME showed no difference from normal populations, except for an increased risk of suicide (Roberts, E. et al. 2016). In common with all others presenting with TFE symptoms, most have no single physical diagnosis. From fifteen separate studies, CBT was effective for reducing fatigue symptoms in ME (Price,

J.R. et al. 2008). In all these instances, ME appeared no different to patients with TFE symptoms reported here, whether ascribed to a clinical entity like ME, chronic fatigue syndrome, or not.

In my experience, what is required for an understanding of TFE symptoms is the in-depth discovery of the psychosocial dynamics; namely, the energy balance factors involved. Ignoring them forces us to focus on psychiatric and physical disease explanations alone.

Some cases, referred to me with palpitation, had an associated, acute onset of fatigue, whereas before, they were normally functioning with normal amounts of perceived energy. I found raised Ebstein Barr antibodies in at least 70% of this group, suggesting (but not proving) an active viral cause. Since EB is an DNA virus, and since tetracyclines inhibit the RNA replication involved in DNA driven processes, I prescribed courses of tetracyclines (usually doxycycline), for those with no obvious antecedent stress. Eighty per-cent of the thirty patients improved, exceeding the expected 20% placebo response rate. These anecdotal findings suggest using a trial of doxycycline in some ME and TFE cases; especially without previous stressful circumstances as a cause for insomnia.

PART THREE

Conclusions

The aim of this treatise has been to explore and explain the clinical, neurophysiological, social and molecular origins of chronic TFE symptoms, and how they might be removed together with any attendant risks.

Both applied stressors and their strain effects need clinical consideration. The stressors faced by patients are multiple and deplete personal cerebral energy. Many involve insecurity, changing situations, fear, and relationship difficulties. Living circumstances vary with socioeconomic background, and have created a health divide. The removal or management of potent stressors is fundamental to improving TFE symptoms or its clinical management.

An important clinical strain effect is the perception of diminishing energy, with patients complaining of tiredness, with some increasing through fatigue to exhaustion. Simultaneously, prone individuals can exhibit pathophysiological changes in blood pressure, heart rate control, immune responses, coagulability and mental health. Some react with panic, anxiety, depression, PTSD, or psychosis, all of which will diminish the ability to cope with everyday issues.

The existence of TFE will often be concurrent with the exacerbation of clinical conditions: angina may occur with less effort; hypertension can become resistant; pneumonia may be less responsive to antibiotics; migraine attacks can become more frequent and psoriasis unresponsive to treatment. Many conditions will resist effective treatment until TFE symptoms are reduced.

Greater cerebral energy expenditure must meet all physical, cognitive, and emotional demands, while homeostasis requires the adequate replenishment of cerebral energy during sleep. To what extent this happens varies between those who respond to stress with insomnia, and those who remain less affected. The effects on sleep – critical to the occurrence of TFE – are likely to have genetic components. Some historic characters have seemed not to require much sleep, regardless of the enormous demands put on them.

The presence of TFE affects daytime wakefulness, clarity of thought, cognitive accuracy, focus, and efficiency, multi-tasking, and global executive functioning. If a discrete part of the brain equivalent to a battery existed, it would be straightforward to postulate its depletion as a cause for TFE symptoms. Since there is no such neurophysiological equivalent, we need another explanation.

Once synthesised, the breaking of one phosphate bond of ATP provides the energy for all cerebral functioning; therefore, ATP depletion might explain tiredness. To ensure survival, however, the brain provides an almost inexhaustible supply of high-energy molecules like ATP, like a tap that is never turned off.

What of neurotransmission? Could a reduction or surfeit of neurotransmitters explain TFE symptoms? For the brain to function normally, an inexhaustible supply of neurotransmitters is also required (some excitatory, some inhibitory). Current evidence suggests that ACh depletion can occur, but only in diseased states like dementia (amyloid, etc.) or cerebral ischaemia from small vessel disease (Jolly, A.A. et al. 2014), perhaps reducing O2 and glucose supply.

Other causes of TFE are intracellular viruses, cell inflammation (multiple sclerosis), and hormone depletion (T4, T3, oestrogen, testosterone, and cortisol) which might deplete cellular ATP (Lawrence, M.S., Sapolsky, RM. 1994).

Without the energy to power and maintain physical health and strength, we would take to our beds, rather than have an active life. The survival of all living organisms depends on having energy available. With reduced energy to cope, adapt or respond to change, we risk a diagnosis of sloth, 'mental breakdown', a 'midlife crisis', 'burn-out syndrome', TATT (Tired All The Time), ME, 'a virus infection' or chronic fatigue syndrome. Such diagnoses, made mostly by exclusion, can suppress the need for further enquiry. Cardiologists and physicians then risk missing the warning symptoms of avoidable catastrophe.

Few doctors, other than psychiatrists, attempt to solve the causes of TFE symptoms by enquiring into the patient's psychosocial problems and the quality of sleep. Doctors busy treating organic disease might prefer social workers or psychiatrists to do this for them. A structured team of counsellors, social workers, cognitive and family therapists, etc., is more likely to serve TFE patients best.

Tiredness, fatigue, and exhaustion can be disease indicators, so physicians investigating patients with TFE symptoms need to address the differential diagnoses. Many are happy to stop after full examination and routine laboratory investigation, but given the known associated risks of TFE, stopping there could disadvantage patients. Not including psychosocial enquiries and asking about sleep could lead to dangerous clinical omission. Not assessing cardiovascular factors in those with TFE symptoms would be to ignore an increased risk for those with hypertension and risk factors for IHD.

Is TFE a physical phenomenon or is it simply perceived as physical? At a global level, not only is tiredness associated with circadian phase, but with the balance of motivational and inhibitory feelings. The more motivated and enthusiastic we become, the more energy we seem to possess; the more dejected and inhibited we feel, the less energy we seem to have. We know that these feelings have a neurochemical basis, driven by the balance of serotonin, dopamine, endorphins, and hormones, as much as by the neurotransmitters AcH, nor-epinephrine and glutamate.

It is clear that neuronal activity produces EEGs of varying power. The power represented by the EEG relates to the amount, intensity, and length of combined cerebral activity. It is impossible at present to link this global activity to either increases or decreases in focal activity, to the type of neurotransmission, or to the synthesis and use of high-energy compounds like ATP and glycogen. The complicated nature of neuronal and neuronal network activity is linked, but far removed from ATP synthesis on one scale, and the generation of EEGs on another. EEGs relate to global functions like consciousness and cognitive activity, but reveal nothing about brain activity at the molecular level.

The causes of TFE at a cellular level could relate to the daytime blocking of neuronal activity (cognition and emotional processing). Various mechanisms might be responsible: activated inhibitory pathways, hyperpolarisation (preventing axonal depolarisation), and changes in plasticity (post-synaptic activation preceding pre-synaptic activation, for instance). These interrupted pathways are likely to be cleared during slow-wave sleep, the result being the restoration of perceived daytime energy. In long-term stress, it is possible that many neuronal pathways remain blocked, and that predominant REM sleep reduces the regeneration of neuronal pathways. In the pathological realm, amyloid in dementia and inflammatory demyelination in multiple sclerosis, both serve as examples of disease related TFE. Also of pathological origin could be small cerebral vessel disease limiting O2 and glucose delivery to astrocytes and other cells.

The new neurophysiological science of 'connectomics', aims to study how the 83 billion brain neurones connect with one another – an extension of Gordon Welchman's, 2nd World War, Traffic Analysis (Welchman, G. 1982). If each neurone connected to only ten others, and one activation tree involved ten neurones, ten billion connections would be possible. If separate depolarisation pathways had a fixed transmission route through the tree of connections (to produce one memory or thought), it might pass through synapses that were fixed, on or off, inhibited or amplified. Indeed, over 100 trillion neuronal connections exist, although some, such as mouse cortex granule cells, possess only four dendritic connections (Caruso, C. 2023). One can hypothesise that each specific pathway through a tree of neurones might be associated with a memory, a thought, an emotive process or be used to make corrections (Nguyen, T.M. et al. 2022). Because every human being has an identifiable personality, character, intelligence, memory, etc., maybe these pathways get set, coming to define the emotive reactions, thoughts, and behaviour patterns typical of each individual.

By comparison, the electrical system of the heart has only one defined pathway. Starting from the sinus node in the right atrium, the depolarisation wavefront passes through both atria to the AV node. Next, the wave stimulates both bundle branches.

Could it be that some people have more pathways expressing sleep and liability to TFE symptoms than others? The benefits of sleep might benefit some more than others. Anatomical fixity of most pathway connections in a mature brain means that connections, although complicated, could be predictable. Because of the many functional synaptic options available within such fixed pathways, the results (thoughts, decisions, emotions, and actions) must be complex and unpredictable ('complicated' and 'complex', as used by Hayek (Hayek, F.A. 1967).

Each demand that excites a cognitive or an emotional response requires neuronal energy to be spent, a derivative of which results in the EEG. The frequency and amplitude of EEG voltages over time, indirectly represent the power spent by cerebral activity. These responses occur within specific time frames, from immediate to delayed. The following considerations apply:

- Immediate cognitive responses can be brief (fast thinking is necessary [Kahneman. 2011]) – arithmetical calculations; deciding whether to catch this bus or the next; deciding whether to stand still or move; deciding whether to reply to a question or remain silent.

- Delayed responses are those that persist unresolved (slow thinking is required [Kahneman. 2011]): whether to effect a change in a relationship; how to solve an ongoing legal or financial problem. These can cause insomnia and daytime TFE. Those with unresolved problems (especially those involving fear or serious concerns about safety and security) can be associated with vivid dreaming or nightmares (increased REM sleep).

Daniel Kahneman (2011), pointed out that when delayed cognition is required, biases can strongly influence thought and decision making. Unresolved stresses cause a constant energy drain. In some, their unresolved presence can add to the perception of tiredness. The more unresolved problems of serious import we have, the more likely insomnia and TFE symptoms are to occur. While on holiday, many ignore their problems, focusing solely on immediate needs. Once TFE symptoms grow, even immediate responses can seem tiresome, aggravating and energy draining. The fewer the background problems, the more enjoyable immediate decision making can become, and the more energy we perceive.

There is evidence for TFE symptoms being a risk factor for both primary and secondary CVS disease, as well as other serious events, yet including TFE symptoms in surveys investigating the prodrome of sudden death is not usual (Marijon, E. et al. 2016)(Keen, S. K., et al. 2021). Psychologists, not cardiologists, have more often made TFE symptoms a point of interest (Appels, A. Orton, F. 1992).

Early recognition of TFE symptoms, especially in patients with established coronary and cerebral artery disease and hypertension (especially those with LVH), could reduce CVS morbidity and mortality. Reducing stressing factors and improving sleep, as well as introducing appropriate cardiac treatment, could reduce CVS morbidity and mortality.

It is important to state that:

- Not every case of cardiac infarction, VF, AF, cerebral infarction or haemorrhage, will be preceded by TFE symptoms.
- Not every case with TFE symptoms will be at risk of CVS catastrophe.

Although TFE symptoms often prove non-specific in clinical diagnosis, they are worthy of physical, psychological, and social enquiry, if the aim is to practise holistic medicine. For prevention, recognition of TFE symptoms is especially important for those with established CVS risk factors (family history, obesity, smoking, diabetes, hyperlipidaemia, athletic unfitness) and evidence of established CVS disease (coronary and cerebral atheroma, and LVH). The prognosis of CVS is driven by these well-defined pathological processes, but often modified by the patient's personal energy considerations.

It is the purpose of this study to attempt an understanding of the mechanisms involved in TFE symptom occurrence. Because this a global cerebral effect, no one factor is likely to explain it. It is obvious from everyday clinical observation that a combination of unresolved chronic stress and sleep deprivation often underlies TFE symptoms. To understand the mechanisms involved, several orders of scale need to be considered, from the molecular level to that of cerebral cellular activation and suppression, to integrating neuronal pathways.

The production of ATP by mitochondria is sensitive to feedback mechanisms related to cellular energy requirements. At the molecular level, ATP, and glycogen utilisation rates, not their generation or storage deficits, are the likely drivers of TFE symptoms (alongside neuronal inhibition). The rapid restoration of perceived energy that soon follows the relief of chronic stress, supports such a conclusion.

The occurrence of TFE symptoms is a global cerebral phenomenon, with no single neurophysiological cause. In theory, it can result from changes at every scale. From molecular alterations in several synaptic transmitters and receptor functions, to complex neuronal activity in and between different cerebral areas, with resulting effects on cognitive and emotional energy expenditure, the quality of sleep, mood change, and other pertinent effects.

At the cellular level, possible mechanisms for TFE symptoms are:

- Diminished neuronal production of transmitters (as found in dementia).
- Altered synaptic plasticity (Diekelmann, S. 2010)(Kuhn, M., et al. 2016). Sleep modulates synaptic plasticity and recalibrates it. In the human brain, sleep deprivation reduces plasticity.
- Reduction in the global numbers of neuronal depolarisations, caused by changes in neurotransmitter production (of ACh, etc.) and plasticity, both of which can inhibit receptor functioning—all of which can be reversed by effective sleep.

At a larger scale:

- Changes in hormone influence (cortisol, T3, T4, oestrogen, melatonin, testosterone, nor-adrenaline).
- Changes in the balance of transmitters that diffuse beyond one synapse: ACh, glutamate, dopamine, serotonin, nor-epinephrine.

- The result of reduced cerebral blood flow with reduced O2 and glucose delivery.

On a global scale:

- Demoralisation and diminished motivation resulting from depression or other mood changes.

This review suggests that reduced ATP availability is an unlikely cause of chronic TFE symptoms. The infinite supply of ATP and neurotransmitters has enabled life and its survival.

Short duration, physical and mental effort, can cause daytime tiredness that is soon recovered by resting for some minutes or hours. A resting brain state (NREM sleep), is necessary to restore the effects of longer term, energy draining effort.

It would seem unlikely that in the normal brain, depletion of ATP, ketones, or glycogen causes chronic TFE symptoms. TFE symptoms are, however, occasionally caused by reduced blood pressure, hypercapnia, and reduced blood glucose or oxygen. Because of the essential nature of these supplies, life would be too vulnerable and would defeat basic evolutionary requirements should any depletion occur.

Synaptic plasticity partly explains the relationship between adequate sleep, defective sleep, and daytime energy in TFE symptom generation. Sleep modulates synaptic plasticity. Both Diekelmann and Kuhn (Diekelmann, S. et al. 2010)(Kuhn, M., et al. (2016), showed that sleep recalibrates synaptic plasticity. In the human brain, sleep deprivation reduces plasticity by increasing synaptic strength (increased current and voltage in post-synaptic neurones). This is associated with an increase in ACh vesicle number, and more ACh released into synaptic clefts. These processes are likely to be involved in the natural history of TFE symptoms.

Sleep can down-scale synaptic strength. Once wakefulness has saturated synapses, sleep can recalibrate them. Certain experiences will saturate synapses so that no further learning can occur from their involvement (Nguyen-Vu, T.D.B. 2017).

Given that ongoing stress and sleep deprivation often combine to cause TFE symptoms, the following global processes are likely involved:

1. The active and stressed daytime brain spends energy and can reach maximal capacitance, because of inhibited synaptic transmission.

2. The function of slow-wave sleep is to reset transmission.

3. Inefficient sleep restoration (an increase in REM and a decrease in NREM sleep) accounts for the various forms of long-term TFE symptoms.

4. The sleep paradox drives inefficient sleep restoration—the greater the stress, the less effective is sleep-related energy regeneration.

The innate global functioning of individual neurotransmission pathways shapes personality, mood, outlook, and behavioural characteristics; all features that predispose to the individual variance of mental and physical energy expenditure.

Although non-specific and varying from person to person, we can easily identify the medical, social, organizational, and relationship causes of greater energy expenditure.

It is likely that the perception of work done, and its relevance to our mission and security in life, determines our energy status, but only for tiredness. Fatigue and exhaustion are more likely the product of ongoing stressful experiences and sleep deprivation.

The perception of reduced energy expenditure, and not a defect in high-energy molecule production, is one cause of TFE symptoms. Comment exists in Xenophon's writings from over 2000 years past. He notes tedium as a cause of TFE, and the need for sleep:

'For not toil, but the tedium of having nothing to do, makes thee long for sleep.'

Xenophon. Memorabilia.

After excluding all treatable physical causes of TFE symptoms (hypothyroidism, Addison's disease, dementia, MS., etc.) and adverse medication effects, clinicians should assess those with remaining psycho-social TFE symptoms for the risk of CVS and other diseases. Those without risk might benefit from counselling (or CBTi) to help remove stressors and allow for increased relaxation and replenishing sleep.

Those with significant risk factors, especially those with evidence of previous cardiac infarction, heart failure, or TIA / stroke, should have more advanced intervention as soon as possible. They should be considered for sleep therapy - a five-day period of frequent sleeping periods – mornings, afternoons and at night, using sedatives to induce sleep. Although non-addictive, sedative antihistamines and antidepressants should be considered first. If cardiac ischaemia, or resistant hypertension is present, benzodiazepines may be indicated. The CVS risk warrants their use, since the risk of addiction is less than that of cardiac infarction, stroke, or death.

I suggest copying the Spartan management of battle fatigue for those able enough: sleep and rest, then physical training to regain fighting fitness. Fitness expands our mental capacity for performance and endurance, perhaps through enthusiasm, self-belief and improved drive. A fit body uses less oxygen and is thus more efficient. How physical exercise effects cerebral energy use is unclear, although there is little doubt that fitness boosts confidence, enthusiasm and can promote replenishing sleep. It can, however, expand glycogen stores in muscles and astrocytes. In ill-health, and recovery from illness or a surgical operation, the opposite occurs. In the exhausted, no energy is available for performance. Those convalescing and recovering from illness achieve minimal performance from the energy they spend. The observation of increased shortness of breath on minimal effort (to gain more oxygen), with little performance achieved, provides some evidence (Fig. 4). For these reasons, we should consider exercise rehabilitation a fundamental intervention for TFE management and relief.

Apparent causative connections between stress and disease can easily fool us, but my viewpoint remains. We must acknowledge possible connections, particularly for those susceptible to pathophysiology (reduced immunity, hypercoagulability, coronary artery disease, and resistant hypertension, etc.). Although some surveys suggest a link between life change and CVS disease, with animal experiments providing circumstantial evidence, no definitive proof of predictability exists. Patients often believe in a connection, and together with their friends and families, will often tell doctors what they think has brought about their medical catastrophe. Extensive reporting of this connection warrants further inquiry.

Postscript

The recognition and management of TFE symptoms could necessitate changes in current medical practice organisation. The provision of longer consultation times and general physicians interested in human demise are both essential. Identifying TFE is easy enough, but more time than usual is often required for its full evaluation and correction. Because TFE can double heart attack risk, these changes are worth making. A political question arises in the UK. How might doctors expand their consultation times and capability to address TFE patient issues—work stress, relationship problems, a lack of resources (money and resources for sleep hygiene), and time off for holidays and healthy pursuits? Should we create dedicated teams for this work if necessary?

A separate important issue is hospital architecture. If patients can rest and sleep well, their prognosis and recovery is likely to improve. Hospital wards often create constant disruption from staff, equipment, and fellow patients' distress, day, and night. The alternative of single room care, more commonly found in private hospitals, also has its problems, although patients prefer this arrangement to Nightingale wards. In private rooms, unwelcome interruptions are fewer. When I worked in Amsterdam, private patients occupied single rooms, part-insured patients shared a double room, and uninsured patients shared a four-bedded room.

The practice of waking patients to give them a sedative drug at a pre-fixed time persists. The need for corporate algorithmic routine, rather than the individualisation of patient care, is responsible. Adequate hospital care for TFE patients with cardiovascular problems requires a team trained in social enquiry and able to manage sleep therapy. Who will sanction their introduction?

With over-specialisation, holistic medicine, of the sort prescribed by Hippocrates and many others, is fading fast. Unfortunately, the focus of corporate medical bureaucracy is maximising patient throughput and not always optimal patient care.

Another issue is doctor and nurse training. Since a doctor's focus is the diagnosis and management of organic disease, many lack an interest in patient welfare, or the time for it. How are we to teach them how best to benefit patients? Doctor–patient continuity, once a key facet of general medicine, has all but disappeared, and with it the early detection (or interest in) chronic fatigue and its relief.

Are we recruiting doctors whose vocation includes caring? Should we recruit medical students, focused only on medical science, rather than patient welfare? With the rules of specialisation now required by the GMC in the UK, specialised rather than broad-based patient management has become mandatory, and dangerous for patients.

As for cardiologists, one would have to recruit not only those capable of implanting pacemakers and passing technical examinations but also those capable of human understanding and sensitivity. Unfortunately, those interested in a technical specialty will not always be those interested in non-specific TFE symptoms.

Although few patients are aware of it, many are suffering at the hands of a medical profession managed by non-clinicians.

Although doctors can identify and control disease, this alone may not satisfy every patient. Those practicing privately in the UK soon discover this truth. Doctors employed by corporations have always had the luxury of pursuing their own practical and academic interests, with little need for patient satisfaction. This has allowed doctors to remain disinterested in their patient's personal problems with a negative impact on those with TFE. If this happened in private practice, patients would withdraw their support, and practices would close.

UK patients now promise, by unwritten contract, that they will not waste their GPs time. They have agreed to be limited to one medical complaint to be discussed at each visit. Also, UK GPs, working limited surgery hours, cannot provide the time to get involved with their patient's marital discord or loss of status. By default, many UK doctors have chosen not to engage with one of the commonest causes of patient demise. Most patients with TFE must remain content to blame spurious conditions like ME or CFS, or unknown viruses for their demise. This situation can have fatal consequences.

The methods outlined within for personal energy assessment and management have proved especially useful for those rejected, or found difficult to diagnose and manage. I should explain that my personal workload - most were tertiary referrals – were cases left unresolved by others (the patient's view, not mine). The reason for failure, on almost every occasion, was not the omission of some exotic blood or scanning test, but a failure to consider the energy exchanges that had led to the patient's demise.

Illustrations

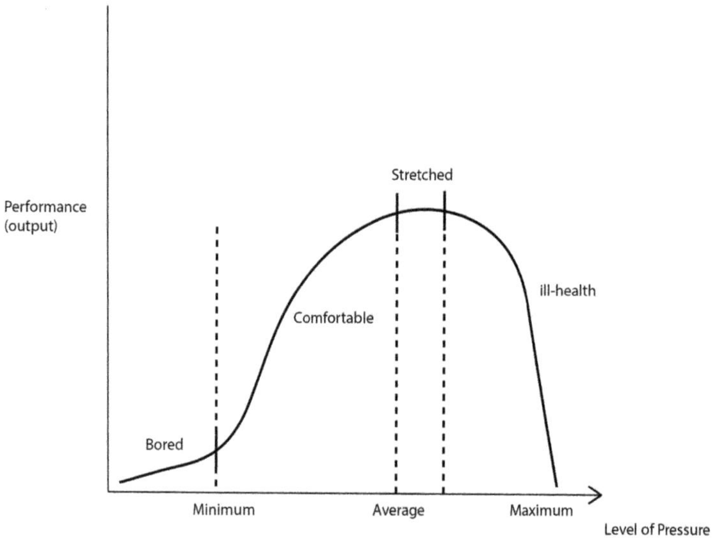

Fig 1. Based on :
(Human Function Curve: Peter Nixon (1979)

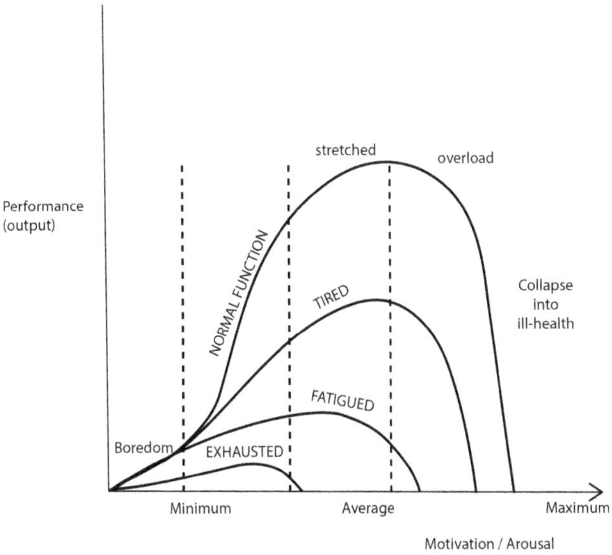

Fig 2.
Human Performance Function in
Normal, Tired, Fatigued, and Exhausted Persons

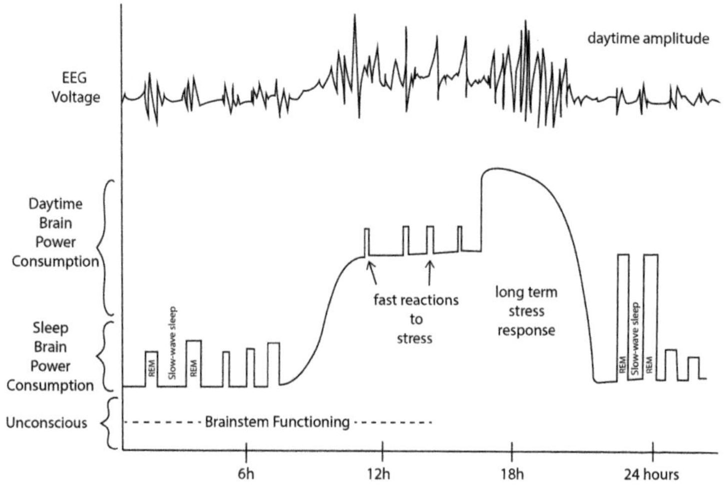

Fig 3.
Schematic for: Brain Power Consumption.
EEG, Phases of Sleep, and Consciousness

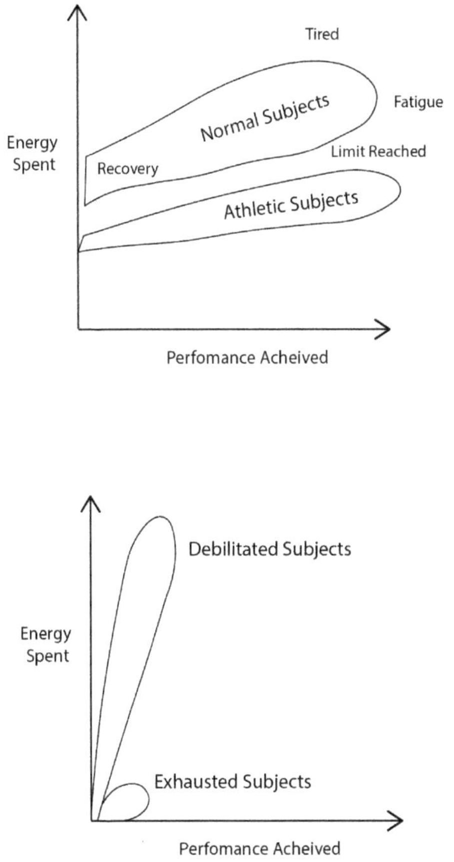

Fig 4.
Performance Acheived versus Perceived Energy Spend in
Normal, Atheltic, Debiliitated (recovery)
and Exhuasted Subjects.

Bibliography

Abromowitz, E.G., Barak. Y. et al. (2010). Hypnotherapy in the Treatment of Chronic Combat-Related PTSD Patients Suffering From Insomnia: A Randomized, Zolpidem-Controlled Clinical Trial. Int. J. of Clin. and Exp. Hypnosis; 56 (3).

Ancoli-Israel, S. (2000). Insomnia in the elderly: a review for the primary care practitioner. Sleep.;23 Suppl 1:S23-30; discussion S36-8.

Ancoli-Israel, S., Liu. L., et al. (2006). Fatigue, sleep and circadian rhythms prior to chemotherapy for breast cancer. Support Care Cancer; 14(3): 201-9.

Anderzen, I., Arnetz. B.B., et al. (1997) Stress and sensitization in children: a controlled prospective psychophysiological study of children exposed to international relocation. J Psychosom Res.;43:259–269.

Appels, A. et al. (1988) Excess fatigue as a precursor of myocardial infarction. Eur Heart J.; 9(7): 758-64.

Appels, A., Orton. F. (1992). Exhaustion as precursor to sudden death. B.J.Clin. Psych.; 31(3): 351-356.

Appels, A, Falger. P.R., Schouten. E.G. (1993) Vital exhaustion as risk indicator for myocardial infarction in women. J Psychosom Res 37, 881–890.

Appels, A., Mulder. P., et al. (1989). Fatigue and heart disease. The association between 'vital exhaustion' and past, present and future heart disease. J. Psychosom. Res.;33(6):727-38.

Archer, Jeffrey. Economic Times: 22/5/2009.

Arendt, J., Aulinas, A. (2022). Physiology of the Pineal Gland and Melatonin. In: Feingold KR, Anawalt B, Blackman MR, et al., editors. Endotext [Internet]. South Dartmouth (MA): MDText.com, Inc.; 2000-. Available from: https://www.ncbi.nlm.nih.gov/books/NBK55097.

Attwell, D, Laughlin. S.B. (2001). An energy budget for signaling in the grey matter of the brain. J Cereb. Blood Flow Metab.; 21(10):1133-45.

Aoun, R., Rawal. H., Attarian. H., Sahni, A. (2019). Impact of traumatic brain injury on sleep: an overview. Nat Sci Sleep. 2019;11:131-140.

Bagheri, B., Meshkini. F. et al. (2016) Life Psychosocial stresses and Coronary Artery Disease. Int J Prev Med.; 7: 106.

Balog, P., Falger. P., et al. (2017) Are vital exhaustion and depression independent risk factors for cardiovascular disease morbidity? Health Psychol.; 36, 740–748.

Bambra, Claire. (2016) The Health Divides. Policy Press.

Beard, G. (1898). Neurasthenia, or nervous exhaustion. The Boston Medical and Surgical Journal 1869; 217-221.

Berchtold, N., Coleman. P.D., et al. (2012). Synaptic genes are extensively downregulated across multiple brain regions in normal aging and Alzheimer's disease. Neurobiol. Aging; 27(6): 1653-1661.

Bernard, C. (1865) Introduction à L'étude de la Médecine Expérimentale. Dover Publications; Mineola, NY, USA.

Bixler, E. O., Vgontzas. A.N., et al. (2005). Excessive daytime sleepiness in a general population sample: the role of sleep apnoea, age, obesity, diabetes, and depression. J Clin Endocrinol Metab.; 90: 4510-5

Blakeman, J.R., Stapleton. S.J. (2018). An integrative review of fatigue experienced by women before and during myocardial infarction. J. Clin. Nurs.; 27(5-6): 906-916).

Blasco-Fontecilla. H., Delgado-Gomez. D., et al. (2012). Can the Holmes-Rahe Social Readjustment Rating Scale (SRRS) Be Used as a Suicide Risk Scale? An Exploratory Study. Arch Suicide Res. 2012;16(1):13–28.

Bonora, M., Patergnani. S.(2012). ATP synthesis and Storage. Purinergic Signal; 8(3):343–357. doi: 10.1007/s11302-012-9305 -8.

Boonstra, T.W., Stins. J.F. (2007). Effects of sleep deprivation on neural functioning: an integrative review. Cell Mol Life Sci; 64(7-8): 934.

Bosma, H., Seigrist. J., et al. (1998). Two alternative job stress models and the risk of coronary heart disease. Am J Public Health 1998;88:68–74.

Boyer, P.D. FASEB J. (1989);3:2164–2178. doi: 10.1096/fasebj.3.10.2526771.

Braley, T.J. & Chervin, R.D. (2010). Fatigue in Multiple Sclerosis: Mechanisms, Evaluation, and Treatment. Sleep; 33(8): 1061-1067.

Breiter, H.C., Rauch. S.L, Kwong. K.K. (1996). Functional magnetic resonance imaging of symptom provocation in obsessive–compulsive disorder. Arch. Gen. Psych. 53, 595–606 (1996).

Bremner, J.D. Brain Imaging in Anxiety Disorders. Expert Rev. Neurotherapeutics 4(2). (2004).

Bremner, J.D., Staib. L., Kaloupek. D. et al. (1999). Neural correlates of exposure to traumatic pictures and sound in Vietnam combat veterans with and without post-traumatic stress disorder: a positron emission tomography study. Biol. Psychiatry 45, 806–816.

Breslin, E., Schans. C van der., et al (1998). Perception of fatigue and quality of life in patients with COPD. Chest; 114(4): 958-64.

Briand, L.A., Gritton. H., et al. (2007) Modulators in concert for cognition: modulator interactions in the prefrontal cortex. Prog Neurobiol.;83:69–91.

Britton, J.W., Frey. L.C., et al., authors (2016); St. Louis EK, Frey LC, editors. Electroencephalography (EEG): An Introductory Text and Atlas of Normal and Abnormal Findings in Adults, Children, and Infants. Chicago: Am. Epilepsy Society.

Bronowski, J. (1975). The Ascent of Man. An Introduction to Human Evolution. BBC Publications. ISBN: 9780563170648.

Brouwer, A. M. et al. Estimating workload using EEG spectral power and ERPs in the n-back task. J. Neural. Eng. 9, 045008 (2012).

Buysse, D.J., Reynolds. C.F. et al. The Pittsburgh Sleep Quality Index: A new instrument for psychiatric practice and research. Psych. Res.: 28(2): 193-213.

Carstairs, V., Morris. R. Deprivation and health in Scotland. Aberdeen: Aberdeen University Press, 1991.

Caruso, C. (Jan 19. 2023). A New Field of Neuroscience Aims to Map Connections in the Brain. Harvard Medical School. News and Research.

Cella, D., Shei-Lai, J., Stone, A. (2011). Self-reported fatigue: one dimension or more? Lessons from the functional assessment of Chronic Illness Therapy (FACT-F) questionnaire. Springer Nature; 19: 1441-1450.

Chamine, I., Atchley. R., Oken. B.S. (2018). Hypnosis intervention effects on sleep outcomes: a systematic review. J Clin Sleep Med.;14(2): 271–283.

Chaput, J.P., Dutil. C., et al. (2020). Sleep timing, sleep consistency, and health in adults: a systematic review. Appl Physiol Nutr Metab.; 45(10 (Suppl. 2)):S232-S247.

Chen, M. (1986). The epidemiology of self-perceived fatigue among adults. Prev Med; 15: 74-81.

Chen, X., Wang. R., Zee. P., et al. (2015).Racial/ethnic differences in sleep disturbances: The Multi-Ethnic Study of Atherosclerosis (MESA). Sleep; 38 (6): 877–888.

Chukwudi, C.U., Good, L. (2016). Interaction of the tetracyclines with double-stranded RNAs of random base sequence: new perspectives on the target and mechanism of action. J. Antibiotics; 69: 622-630.

Chukwudi, C.U., Good, L. (2019). Doxycycline inhibits pre-rRNA processing and mature rRNA formation in E.coli. J. Antibiotics (Tokyo); 72(4):225-236.

Citri, A., Malenka, R.C. (2008). Synaptic Plasticity: Multiple Forms, Functions and Mechanisms. Neuropsychopharmacology; 33: 18-41.

Clark, A., Strandberg-Larsen. K., et al.(2015) Psychosocial risk factors for hospitalisation and death from chronic obstructive pulmonary disease: A prospective cohort study. COPD 12, 190–198.

Cleare, A.J. 2003) The neuroendocrinology of chronic fatigue syndrome. Endocr Rev. 2003;24:236–52.

Colrain, I.M., Nicholas, C.L., Baker, F.C. (2014). Alcohol and the Seeping Brain. Handbook of Clin Neurol.;125:415–431.

Cook, D.B., et al. (2007). Functional neuroimaging correlates of mental fatigue induced by cognition among chronic fatigue syndrome patients and controls. NeuroImage, doi:10.1016/j.neuroimage.2007.02.033.

Costello, R.B., et al. (2014). The effectiveness of melatonin for promoting healthy sleep: a rapid evidence assessment of the literature. Nutrition. Journal; 13: 106.

Cryer, P. E. (2007). Hypoglycaemia, functional brain failure, and brain death. J. Clin. Invest.; 117(4):868-870.

Dai, X., Zhou. E. (2021). Molecular resolution of a behavioural paradox: sleep and arousal are regulated by distinct acetylcholine receptors in different neuronal types in Drosiphila. Sleep; 44(7) zsab017.

Dasari, D., Shou, G. & Ding, L. ICA-derived EEG correlates to mental fatigue, effort, and workload in a realistically simulated air traffic control task. Front. Neurosci. 11, 297 (2017).

DEFRA.(2022) Statistical Digest of Rural England. Crime.

de Faire, U., Theorell, T. (1976). Life Changes and Myocardial Infarction. Scand. J. Soc. Med; 4:115-122.

de Rijk, A. E., Schreurs, K. M., Bensing J. M. (1999).What is behind "I'm so tired"? Fatigue experiences and their relations to the quality and quantity of external stimulation. J. Psychosom. Res.;47(6):509–523.

Dewa, L.H., Hassan, L. et al (2017). Trouble sleeping inside: a cross-sectional study of the prevalence and associated risk factors of insomnia in adult prison populations in England. Sleep Med.; 32: 129-136.

Diamond, D.M, Fleshner, M., Ingersoll, N,. Rose, G.M. (1996). Psychological stress impairs spatial working memory: relevance to electrophysiological studies of hippocampal function. Behav. Neurosci. 110, 661–672.

Dickens, Charles.(1837). Pickwick Papers. Chapman and Hall. London

Dickens, Charles. (1850) David Copperfield.

Diekelmann, S. & Born, J. (2010). The memory function of sleep. Nat. Rev. Neurosci.; 11: 114–126.

Dighton, D.H. (1974). Sinus Bradycardia. BHJ; 36:791-797.

Dighton, D.H. (2023). The NHS. Our Sick Sacred Cow. Medicause.

Dighton, D.H. (2024) The Art & Science of Medical Practice. MediCause.

Digman, J.M. (1990). Personality structure: Emergence of the five-factor model. Annual Review of Psychology. 1990; 41:417-440.

DSM-5 Diagnostic Criteria for PTSD. (Center for Substance Abuse Treatment (US). Trauma-Informed Care in Behavioral Health Services. Rockville (MD): Substance Abuse and Mental Health Services Administration (US); 2014. (Treatment Improvement Protocol (TIP) Series, No. 57.)

du Bois-Reymond, E. (1848–1884). Untersuchungen über thierische Electricität. Vol. 2 Berlin: Reimer.

Dunlop, B.W., Mayberg, H.S. (2017). Neuroimaging Advances for Depression. Cerebrum; 2017 Nov 1; 2017:cer-16-17.

Dunn, J. Grider, M.H. (2023). Physiology, Adenosine Triphosphate. StatPearls (Internet).

Duranni, D., Idress, R., et al. (2022). Vitamin B6: A new approach to lowering anxiety, and depression? Ann. Med. Surg. (Lond); 82:104663. doi: 10.1016/j.amsu.2022.104663).

Dutheil, F., Danini, B., et al. (2021) Effects of a short daytime nap on the cognitive performance: A systematic review and meta-analysis. International Journal of Environmental Research and Public Health, 18(19), 10212

Elmquest, Jen. (2017) Relationship Reset. ISBN: 978-0997458107.

Eames, M., ben Shlomo, Y., Marmot, M.G. (1993). Social deprivation and premature mortality: regional comparison across England. BMJ; 307 (6912): 1097-1102.

Edinger, J.D., Bonnet, M.H., Bootzin, R.R. (2024). Derivation of research diagnostic criteria for insomnia: report of an American Academy of Sleep Medicine Work Group. Sleep.;27(8):1567–15 96.

Elenkov, I. J. (2008). Neurohormonal-cytokine interactions: implications for inflammation, common human diseases and well-being. Neurochem. Int. 52, 40–51).

Elkins, G, Johnson. A, et al. (2013). A pilot investigation of guided self-hypnosis in the treatment of hot flashes among postmenopausal women. Int J Clin Exp Hypn.; 61(3): 342–350.

Elwert, F., and Christakis, N.A. (2008). The Effect of Widowhood on Mortality by the Causes of Death of Both Spouses. Am. J. Public Health; 98(11): 2092-2098.

Faber, P.L., Lehmann, D. et al. (2012). EEG source imaging during two Qigong meditations. Cogn. Process: 13(3): 255-65).

Feynman, R., Wilczek, F. (2020). The Character of Physical Law. MIT Press.

Finkelstein, G. (2015). Editorial. Mechanical Neuroscience: Emil du Bois-Reymond;s Innovations in Theory and Practice. Front. Syst. Neurosci.; 9: 133.

Fischler, B., Cluydts, R. et al. (1997). Generalized anxiety disorder in chronic fatigue syndrome. Acta. Psych. Scand.; 95(5):405-413.

Fitzgerald, S.P., Pope, K.J. (2004). Cognitive tasks augment gamma EEG power. Clin Neorophys.; 115: 1802-1809.

Ford, D.E., Kamerow, D.B. (1989). Epidemiologic Study of Sleep Disturbance and Psychiatric Disorders. An Opportunity for Prevention? JAMA; 262(11): 1479-1484.

Frank, M.G, Heller, H.C.(2019) The Function(s) of Sleep. Handb Exp Pharmacol.; 253:3-34.

Frestad, D, Prescott, E. (2017) Vital exhaustion and coronary heart disease risk: A systematic review and meta-analysis. Psychosom Med 79, 260–272.

Freud, S. (1900). The interpretation of dreams. In The Standard Edition of the Complete Works of Sigmund Freud, Vol. 4, 5, ed. Strachey J. (London: Hogarth Press).

Freud, Sigmund. (1901). On Dreams. The Standard Edition of the Complete Psychological Works of Sigmund Freud, Volume V (1900-1901): The Interpretation of Dreams (Second Part) and On Dreams, 629-686.

Freiberg, A.S. (2020). Why We Sleep: A Hypothesis for an Ultimate or Evolutionary Origin of Slee and Physiological Rhythms. J. Circadian Rhythms; 18(2). doi: 10.5334/jcr.189.

Friedman, M., Rosenman, R.H., Carroll. V. (1958) Changes in the serum cholesterol and blood clotting time in men subjected to cyclical variations in occupational stress. Circulation;17: 852–61.

Friedman, M., Rosenman, R. (1959). Association of specific overt behaviour pattern with blood and cardiovascular findings. Journal of the American Medical Association. 169 (12): 1286–1296.

Fujita, N. (1956). Pharmacological Study on Electrical Activity and Oxygen Consumption of Brain Cortex. J Jap Pharm; 5: 151-173.

Gallacher, J.E.J., Sweetnam, P.M. et al. (2003). Is Type A Behaviour Really a Trigger for CHD Events? Psychosom. Med. 65(3): 339-46.

Gastel, J.A., Rosenboom, P.H. et al. (1998). Melatonin production: proteasomal proteolysis in serotonin N-acetyltransferase regulation. Science (New York, NY); 279(5355):1358–60.

Gottman, J. The Gottman Institute. www.gottman.com/blog/manage-conflict-using

Gottesmann, C. 2012). GABA mechanisms and sleep. Neuroscience. 2002;111(2):231-9.

Gurvits, T.G., Shenton, M.R., Hokama, H. et al. (1996). Magnetic resonance imaging study of hippocampal volume in chronic combat-related post-traumatic stress disorder. Biol. Psych. 40, 192–199.

Habert, R., Claude Bernard. The Founder of Modern Medicine. Cells (2022); 11(10):1702.

Hagins, M., States, R. et al. (2013). Effectiveness of Yoga for Hypertension: Systematic Review and Meta-Analysis. Evidence-based Complementary and Alternative medicine. Vol. 2013: issue 1/ 64983.

Halassa, M.M., Florian, C. et al.(2009). Astrocytic modulation of sleep homeostasis and cognitive consequences of sleep loss. Neuron; 61(2):213-9.

Hall, Calvin. (1971). The Personality of a Child Molester. An Analysis of Dreams. Routledge. ISBN: 9781315133805.

Hann, D. M., Jacobsen, P. B., et al. (1998) Measurement of fatigue in cancer patients: development and validation of the Fatigue Symptom Inventory. Qual. Life Res;7(4):301–310.

Hanson, G.K. (2001). Immune Mechanisms in Atherosclerosis. Arteriosclerosis, Thrombosis and Vascular Biol.; 21(12).

Hao, J. Oertner, T.G. (2012). Depolarization gates spine calcium transients and spike-timing-dependent potentiation. Current Opinion in Neurobiology; 22(3): 509-515).

Harnett, M.T., Makara, J.K. et al. (2013). Synaptic amplification by dendritic spines enhances input cooperativity. Nature.; 491 (7425):599-602.

Harris, J. J., Jolivet, R., Attwell. D. (2012). Synaptic energy use and supply. Neuron 75, 762–777. 10.1016/j.neuron.2012.08.019.

Hasler, G. (2010). Pathophysiology of Depression: Do we have any solid evidence of interest to clinicians? World Psychiatry; 9(3):155-161.

Hayek, F.A. (1967). The theory of complex phenomena. Studies in philosophy, politics and economics. University of Chicago Press, Chicago.

Haynes, S.G., Feinleib, M. (1980). Women, work and coronary heart disease: prospective findings from the Framingham heart study. Am. J. Public Health; 70(2):133-41.

Hebb, D.O. (1949). The Organisation of Behaviour. A Neuropsychological Theory. (Routledge).

Hernandez-Aceituno, A., Guallar-Castillon, P., et al.(2019). Association between sleep characteristics and antihypertensive treatment in older adults. Geriatrics and Gerontology International . 2019;19(6):537–540

Herrnstein, R., and Murray, C.A.(1994): 'The Bell Curve'. Intelligence and Class Structure in American Life). Free Press.

Hilditch, C.J., McHill, A.W (2019). Sleep inertia: current insights. Nat Sci Sleep.;11:155-165.

Hoel, Erik. (2021).The overfitted brain: dreams evolved to assist generalisation. Patterns (n/Y); 2(5): 100244.

Holbrook, A., Crowther, R., et al. (2001). The role of benzodiazepines in the treatment of insomnia: meta-analysis of benzodiazepine use in the treatment of insomnia. J Am Geriatr Soc.;49(6):824-6.

Holm, A., Lukander, K., Korpela, J., Sallinen, M. & Muller, K. M. I. (2009). Estimating brain load from the EEG. Sci. World J. 9, 639–651.

Homer. The Odyssey. Book iv. Ryerson Univ. Toronto. 2022.

Huber, R. et al. (2012). Human cortical excitability increases with time awake. Cereb. Cortex; 23: 332–338.

Hublin, C., Kaprio, M. et al (1996). Daytime sleepiness in an adult, Finnish population. J. Int. Med.; 239:417-423.

Hwang, J-H., Lee, J-S. et al. (2023). Evaluation of viral infection as an etiology of ME/CFS: a systematic review and meta-analysis. J. Transl. Med.; 21: 763.

Institute of Medicine (US) Committee on Sleep Medicine and Research (2006). Sleep Disorders and Sleep Deprivation: An Unmet Public Health Problem. Colten, H.R, Altevogt, B. M, editors. National Academies Press (US); Washington (DC).

Irwin, M.R. (2015) Why sleep is important for health: a psychoneuroimmunology perspective. Annual Rev. Psychol.; 66:143–172.

Islamoska, S., Ishtiak-Ahmed, K. (2019).Vital Exhaustion and Incidence of Dementia: Results from the Copenhagen City Heart Study. J. Alzheimers Disease; 67(1):369-379.

Iversen, L., Strandberg-Larsen, K., et al. (2012) Psychosocial risk factors, weight changes and risk of obesity: The Copenhagen City Heart Study. Eur J Epidemiol 27, 119–130.

Janssens, K.A., Zijlema, W.L. et al (2015). Mood and Anxiety Disorders in Chronic Fatigue Syndrome, Fibromyalgia, and Irritable Bowel Syndrome: Results From the LifeLines Cohort Study. Psychosom. Med.; 77(4):449-57.

Jarman, B. (1983) Identification of underprivileged areas. BMJ;286:1705-9.

Javaheri, S., Redline, S. (2017). Insomnia and Risk of cardiovascular Disease. Chest; 152(2): 435-444.

Jevning, R., Wallace, R.K., et al. (1992). The physiology of meditation: a review. A wakeful hypometabolic integrated response. Neuroscience and Biobehavioural Reviews; 16(3): 415-424.

Jolly, A.A., Brown, R.B., et al. (2024). Are central and systemic inflammation associated with fatigue in cerebral small vessel disease? Int. J. Stroke; 19(6): 705-713.

Joshi, A.M. et al. (2024). Therapeutic Role of Yoga in Hypertension. World J. Methodology; 14(1): 90127.

Kahneman, Daniel. Thinking Fast and Slow (2011). Penguin Books.

Kaira, S., Sahay, R. (2018). Diabetes Fatigue Syndrome. Diabetes Ther.; 9(4): 1421-1429.

Kandola, Aaron. (2024). How Can I Get to Sleep Easily? Medical News Today (www.medicalnewstoday.com/articles/322928.

Kaneita, Y., Ohida, T., et al. (2005). Excessive daytime sleepiness among the Japanese general population. J Epidemiol.;15:1-8.

Karakurt, P. & Ünsal, A. (2013). Fatigue, anxiety and depression levels, activities of daily living of patients with chronic obstructive pulmonary disease. International Journal of Nursing Practice, 19(2), 221–231.

Karndar, B.B., Needham, D.M., Collop, N.A. (2012). Sleep Deprivation in Critical Illness: Its Role in Physical and Psychological Recovery. J Intensive Care Med.; 27(2):97–111. doi: 10.1177/0885066610394322.

Katafuchi, T., Kondo, T., et al. (2005). Enhanced expression of brain interferon-alpha and serotonin transporter in immunologically induced fatigue in rats. *Eur J Neurosci. ;22:2817–2826. doi: 10.1111/j.1460-9568.2005.04478.x.*

Kataoka, Y., Yamato., et al. (2013). Neuroinflammation in animal models of fatigue. *Adv Neuroimmune Biol. 2013;4:237–244.*

Katyal, S., Goldin, P. (2021). Alpha and theta oscillations are inversely related to progressive levels of meditation depth. Neurosci. Conscious. 2021(1):niab042.

Katz, B. (1969) The Release of Neural Transmitter Substances. Liverpool Univ. Press; Liverpool.

Kaufmann, C.N., Canham, S.L., et al. (2013). Insomnia and health services utilization in middle-aged and older adults: Results from the Health and Retirement Study. The Journals of Gerontology Series A: Biological Sciences and Medical Sciences.; 68:1512–1517.

Kawachi, I., Sparrow, D., et al. (1998). Prospective study of a self-report Type-A Scale and Risk of Coronary Heart Disease. Circulation; 98(5): 405-412.

Keen, S.K., Masoudi, E.A., et al. (2012). Symptoms prior to sudden death. Resus Plus; 5:100078

Kilduff, T.S., Krilowicz, B. et al (1993). Sleep and Mammalian Hibernation: Homologous Adaptations and Homologous Processes? Sleep; 16(4): 372-386.

Kim, M.C., Fricchione, E.N. et al. (2020). Electroencephalogram oscillations and the spectrogram in monitoring anaesthesia. BJA. Education; 20(5): 166-172.)

Kim, S.C., Lee, M.H., et al. (2014). The Effect of Alpha Rhythm Sleep on EEG Activity and Individual's Attention. J. Phys. Ther. Sci.; 25(12): 1515-1518.

King, C.R., Knutson, K.L., et al. (2008). Short sleep duration and incident coronary artery calcification. JAMA.;300(24):2859 –2866.

Kivimäki, M., Jokela, M., et al. (2015). Long working hours and risk of coronary heart disease and stroke: a systematic review and meta-analysis of published and unpublished data for 603,838 individuals. Lancet; 386 (10005): 1739-1746.

Koopman, A. D. M., Beulens, J. W., et al. (2020) Prevalence of insomnia (symptoms) in T2D and association with metabolic parameters and glycemic control: meta-analysis. The Journal of Clinical Endocrinology & Metabolism;105(3):614–643.

Kop, W.J., Appels, A.P. et al. (1994) Vital exhaustion predicts new cardiac events after successful coronary angioplasty. Psychosom Med.;56(4):281-7.

Kop, W. (2012) Somatic depressive symptoms, vital exhaustion, and fatigue: Divergent validity of overlapping constructs. Psychosom Med 74, 442–445.

Krizanova, O., Babula, P., Pacak, K. (2016). Stress, catecholaminergic system and cancer. Stress 19, 419–428).

Kuczewski, N., Azteria, E. et al. (2005). Acetylcholine modulates cortical synaptic transmission via different muscarinic receptors, as studied with receptor knockout mice. J. Physiology; 566 (Pt 3: 907-919.

Kuhn, M., Wolf, E. et al. (2016). Sleep calibrates homeostatic and associative synaptic plasticity in the human cortex. Nature Communications 7: 12455.

Labarca, G, Reyes, T, et al. (2018). CPAP in patients with obstructive sleep apnea and type 2 diabetes mellitus: Systematic review and meta-analysis. Clin. Respir. J.;12(8):2361-2368.

Lawrence, M.S., Sapolsky, RM. (1994). Glucocorticoids accelerate ATP loss following metabolic insults in cultured hippocampal neurons. Brain Res. 646, 303–306.

Lee, J., Hong, Y., et al. (2021). Prevalence of Insomnia in Various Industries and Associated Demographic Factors in Night-Shift Workers Using Workers' Specific Health Examination Data. Int. J. Environ. Res. Public Health; 18(13):6902.

Lehrskov, L.L., Dorph, E. et al. (2018). The Role of IL-1 in Post-Prandial Fatigue. Mol. Met.; 12: 107-112.

Leuzinger, W. (1969). Structure and function of acetylcholinesterase. Prog Brain Res. 1969; 31:241-5.

Lewis, G., Wessely, S. (1992). The epidemiology of fatigue: more questions than answers. J. Epidemiology and Community Health; 46:92-97.

Leyland, A., Rowse, G., Emerson, L-M.(2019). Experimental effects of mindfulness inductions on self-regulation: systematic review and meta-analysis. Emotion;19:108–22.

Lichstein, K.L., Wilson, N.M., et al.(1994). Daytime sleepiness in insomnia: behavioural, biological and subjective indices. Sleep; 17(8):693-702.

Liedloff, Jean. (1975). The Continuum Concept. Penguin Books. 1989.

Lin, W. Q., Jing, M. J. et al. (2015). Factors associated with fatigue among men aged 45 and older: A cross-sectional study. International Journal of Environmental Research and Public Health, 12(9), 10897–10909.

Liu, D., Yu, C. et al (2022). The Association between Hypertension and Insomnia: A Bidirectional Meta-Analysis of Prospective Cohort Studies. Int. J. Hypertension; 2022:4476905.

Liu, X., Zhang, H. et al. (2024). EEG-based major depressive disorder recognition by neural oscillation and asymmetry. Front. Neuroscience; 18: 1362111.

Liu, Y.Z., Wang. Y.X. et al. (2017) Inflammation: The Common Pathway of Stress-Related Diseases. Front. Hum. Neuroscience; 11:316.

Llorente-Folch, I., Rueda., C.B. (2015). The regulation of neuronal mitochondrial metabolism by calcium. J. Physiology; 593(16):3447-62. doi: 10.1113/JP270254.

Loge, J. H., Ekeberg, O., Kaasa, S. (1998) Fatigue in the general Norwegian population: normative data and associations. J Psychosom. Res.;45(1):53–65.

Long, D., Mackenbach, J.P., Klokgieters, S. et al. Widening educational inequalities in mortality in more recent birth cohorts: a study of 14 European countries. J Epidemiol Community Health ; 77: 400-408.

Løvlien, M., Johansson, I. et al. (2009). Early warning signs of an acute myocardial infarction and their influence on symptoms during the acute phase, with comparisons by gender. Gender Med.; 6(3): 444-453.

Lysakowski, A., Wainer, B.H., et al.(1989. An atlas of the regional and laminar distribution of choline acetyltransferase immunoreactivity in rat cerebral cortex. Neuroscience.; 28:291–336.

Macefield, G., Gandevia, S.C., Burke. D.(1989). Conduction velocities in muscle and cutaneous afferents in the upper and lower limbs of human subjects. Brain; 112(6): 1519-1532.

Maes, M., Mihaylova, I. et al. (2005). Decreased dehydroepiandrosterone sulfate but normal insulin-like growth factor in chronic fatigue syndrome (CFS): relevance for the inflammatory response in CFS. Neuro Endocrinol Lett. 2005;26:487–92).

Magowan, S.R. (2017). Approaching Sleep and Dreams in Early Greek Thought. PhD thesis submission. Univ. London.

Malivanova, S.D. (1968). Cholinesterase activity of the nervous system apparatus and myocardium in rabbits heart during experimental diphtheritic myocarditis. Doklady Academi Nauk. SSSR; 178: 213.

Marijon, E., Uy-Avenado, A. et al. (2016). Warning Symptoms Are Associated With Survival From Sudden Cardiac Arrest. Ann. Int. Med.; 164(1): 23-29.

Marmot, M.G., Smith, G.D. et al. (1997). Socio-economic Differentials in Health. J. Health Psych; 2(3).

Marmot, M.G., Bosma, H. et al (1997). Contribution of job control and other risk factors to social variations in coronary heart disease incidence. Lancet; 350(9073):235-9).

Mascetti, G.G. (2016). Unihemispheric sleep and asymmetrical sleep: behavioral, neurophysiological, and functional perspectives. Nat. Sci. Sleep; 8: 221-238.

Matsui, T., Omuro, H. et al. (2017). Astrocytic glycogen-derived lactate fuels the brain during exhaustive exercise to maintain endurance capacity. Proc. Nat. Acad. Sci. of the USA (PNAS); 114 (24) 6358-6363.

McDougall, W. (1932). Of the words character and personality. Character and Personality; 1: 3–16.

Meier-Ewert, H.K., Ridker, P.M., Rifai, N. (2004). Effect of sleep loss on C-reactive protein, an inflammatory marker of cardiovascular risk. J Am Coll Cardiol.;43(4):678–683.

MedlinePlus. National Library of Medicine. Medical Encyclopedia: blood gases.

Memar, P., Faradji, F. (2018). A Novel Multi-Class EEG-Based Sleep Stage Classification System. IEEE Trans Neural Syst Rehabil Eng. ;26(1):84-95.

Michielsen, H. J., De Vries, J., & Van Heck, G. L. (2003). Psychometric qualities of a brief self-rated fatigue measure the fatigue assessment scale. Journal of Psychosomatic Research, 54, 345–352.

Miller, A. H., Maletic, V., Raison, C. L. (2009). Inflammation and its discontents: the role of cytokines in the pathophysiology of major depression. Biol. Psychiatry 65, 732–741.

Mills, J.N., Minors, D.S., Waterhouse, J.M. (1974). The circadian rhythms of human subjects without timepieces or indication of the alternation of day and night. J. Physiology; 240(3): 567-594.

Mira López, E. (1943). Psychiatry in war. Norton.

Modig, K., Talbäck, M. et al. (2017). Payback time? Influence of having children on mortality in old age. Epidem. & Community Health; 71(5): 424-430.

Morin, C.M., Culbert, J.P., Schwartz, S.M. (1994). Non-pharmacological interventions for insomnia: a meta-analysis of treatment efficacy. The American Journal of Psychiatry; 151(8):1172–1180.

Morin, C.M., Vallières, A, et al. (2009) Cognitive behavioral therapy, singly and combined with medication, for persistent insomnia: a randomized controlled trial. JAMA; 301 (19): 2005–2015.

Mostofsky, E., Maclure, M. et al (2012). Risk of acute myocardial infarction after the death of a significant person in one's life: the Determinants of Myocardial Infarction Onset Study. Circulation; 125(3): 491-496.

Murillo-Rodríguez, E., Arias-Carrión, O., et al. (2009) Mechanisms of sleep-wake cycle modulation. CNS Neurol Disord Drug Targets.;8(4):245-53.

Muramatsu, I., Masuoka, T., et al. (2018). A New Aspect of Cholinergic Transmission in the Central Nervous System. In: Akaike, A., Shimohama, S., Misu, Y., editors. Nicotinic Acetylcholine Receptor Signaling in Neuroprotection [Internet]. Springer; Singapore: Apr 4, 2018. pp. 45– 58.

Muscio, B. Is a fatigue test possible? Br. Psychology 1921; 12: 31-46.

Nadrowski, P., Chudek J., et al. (2016). Associations between cardiovascular disease risk factors and IL-6 and hsCRP levels in the elderly. Exp. Gerontol. 85, 112–117.

Nakamoto, R.K., Scanlon, J.A., Baylis, Al-Shawi, M.K. (2008). The Rotary Mechanism of the ATP Synthase. Arch. Biochem. Biophys.; 476(1):43–50.

Nelson, T., Zhang. L-X. et al. (2021). Brainstem Abnormalities in Myalgic Encephalomyelitis/Chronic Fatigue Syndrome: A Scoping Review and Evaluation of Magnetic Resonance Imaging Findings. Front. Neuro.;12:769511.

Nguyen-Vu, T.D.B., Zhao, G.Q., et al.(2017). A saturation hypothesis to explain both advanced and impaired learning with enhanced plasticity. eLife. Feb24;6:e20147

Nguyen, T.M., Thomas, L.A., et al. (2023). Structured Cerebellar Activity Supports Resilient Pattern Seperation. Nature; 613: 543 – 549.

Niwa, Y. et al (2018). Muscarinic acetylcholine receptors CHrm1 and Chrm3 are essential for REM sleep. Cell Rep. 24(9):2231-2247.e4

Nixon, P.G. (1976). The Human Function Curve. With special reference to cardiovascular disorders. Practitioner; 217(1302):935-44.

Nixon. P.G. (1982). The human function curve – a paradigm for our times. Activitas Nervosa Superior, Suppl. 3 (part 1): 130-133.

Noji, H., Yasuda, R., Yoshida, M., Kinosita, K. Direct observation of the rotation of F1-ATPase. Nature. 1997; 386:299–302.

NSC. US National Safety Council (nsc.org). Cost of Fatigue at Work. (2025). Headquarters: Itasca, Illinois. US.

Oakley, Anne. (1990). Housewife. High Value. Low Cost. Penguin.

Office for National Statistics (England). (2020). Socioeconomic Inequalities in Avoidable Mortality.

Öz. G., Seaquist. E.R., et al. (2007). Human Brain Glycogen Content and Metabolism: Implications on itd Role in Brain Energy Metabolism. Am. J. Physiol. Endocrinol. Metab.; 292(3): E946-51.

Öz, G., DiNuzzo, M., et al. (2015). Revisiting Glycogen Content in the Human Brain. Neurochem. Res.; 40(12):2473-81.

Pallesen, S., Nordhus, I.H., et al. (2007). Prevalence and risk factors of subjective sleepiness in the general adult population. Sleep;30:619-24.

Parikh, V., Man, K., et al. (2008). Glutamatergic contributions to nicotinic acetylcholine receptor agonist-evoked cholinergic transients in the prefrontal cortex. J Neurosci.;28:3769–3780.

Partinen, M., Putkonen, P.T.S., et al. (1982). Sleep disorders in relation to coronary heart disease. Acta Medica Scandinavica, 211(S660), pp.69-83.

Partinen, M., Eskelinen, L., Tuomi, K. (1984). Complaints of insomnia in different occupations. Scand. J. Work Environ. Health.;10: 467–469.

Patel, A.K., Reddy, V. (2024). Physiology, Sleep Stages. [Updated 2024 Jan 26]. In: StatPearls [Internet]. Treasure Island (FL):

StatPearls Publishing; 2025 Jan-. Available from: https://www.ncbi.nlm.nih.gov/books/NBK526132/

Pawlikowska, T., Chalder, T. et al. (1994). Population based study of fatigue and psychological distress. BMJ 308 (1994), pp. 763- 766.

Pedersen, J., Lund, R., et al. (2016) Psychosocial risk factors for the metabolic syndrome: A prospective cohort study. Int. J. Cardiol.; 215: 41–46.

Peever, J., Fuller, P.M. The Biology of REM Sleep. Curr Biol.; 27(22):R1237-R1248.

Piciotto, M.R., Higley, M.J., Mineur, Y.S. (2012). Acetylcholine as a neuromodulator: cholinergic signaling shapes nervous system function and behaviour. Neuron; 76(1):116–129.

Pierce, B. L., Ballard-Barbash, R., et al. (2009). Elevated biomarkers of inflammation are associated with reduced survival among breast cancer patients. J. Clin. Oncol. 27, 3437–3444).

Plato. Phaedrus. 230d. Michael Marder (2012. Nov. 26). The Philosopher's Plant 1.0: Plato's Plane Tree. Project Syndicate.

Price, J.R., Mitchell, E., et al.(2008). Cognitive behaviour therapy for chronic fatigue syndrome in adults. Cochrane Database Syst. Rev.; (3):CD001027.

Puma, S., Matton, N., et al. (2018) Using theta and alpha band power to assess cognitive workload in multitasking environments. Int. J. Psychophysiol. 123, 111–120).

Gabriela Quinlan, Mehmet Ali Döke, et al. (2023) Carbohydrate nutrition associated with health of overwintering honey bees. Journal of Insect Science; 23 (6): 16. doi: 10.1093/jisesa/iead084.

Ragland, D.R., Brand, R.J. (1988). Type a Behavior and Mortality from Coronary Heart Disease.
N. Engl. J Med.; 318:65-69.

Ragland, D.R., Brand. R.J. (1988). Coronary heart disease mortality in the Western Collaborative Group Study. Follow-up experience of 22 years. Am. J. Epidem. 127(3):462-75.

Rampersad, S., Tennant. P. (2018). Replication and Expression Strategies of viruses. Viruses; 30: 55-82.

Redelmeier, D.A., Greenwald, J.A. (2007) Competing risks of mortality with marathons: retrospective analysis. BMJ; 335(7633): 1275-1277.

Rees, W.D. & Lutkins, S.G. (1967). Mortality of Bereavement. BMJ; 4: 13-16.

Riemann, D. (2020). Hyperarousal and insomnia: state of the science. Sleep Med Rev. 2010;14(1):17.

Roberts, E., Wessley, S., et al. (2016). Mortality of people with chronic fatigue syndrome: a retrospective cohort study in England and Wales from the South London and Maudsley NHS Foundation Trust Biomedical Research Centre (SLaM BRC) Clinical Record Interactive Search (CRIS) Register. Lancet; 387(10028):1638-43.

Rodenbeck, A., Cohrs S., et al. (2003). The sleep-improving effects of doxepin are paralleled by a normalized plasma cortisol secretion in primary insomnia. A placebo-controlled, double-blind, randomized, cross-over study followed by an open treatment over 3 weeks. Psychopharmacology (Berl) 2003;170(4):423–428.

Rosekind, M. R., Smith, R. M., et al. (1995). Alertness management: strategic naps in operational settings. Journal of Sleep Research, 4(S2), 62–66.

Roy, C.S., Sherringham, C.S. et al. (1890). On the Regulation of Blood-Supply to the Brain. J Physiol. Jan;11(1-2):85-158.17.

Salleh, M. R. (2008). Life Event, Stress and Illness. Malaysian J. Med. Sci. 15(4):9–18.

Sargent, W. (1967) The Unquiet Mind. ISBN: 0 330 02635 6. Heinemann.

Sartar, M., Parikh, V., Howe, W.M.(2009). Phasic acetylcholine release and the volume transmission hypothesis: time to move on. Nat Rev Neurosci.;10(5):383–390.

Saunders, A., Granger. A.J., et al. (2015). Corelease of acetylcholine and GABA from cholinergic forebrain neurones. eLife 4:e06412.

Schmitt, L.I., Sims, R.E. et al. (2012). Wakefulness Affects Synaptic and Network Activity by Increasing Extracellular Astrocyte-Derived Adenosine. J. of Neuroscience; 32(13):4417-4425.

Schuitemaker, G.E., et al. (2004). Assessment of vital exhaustion and identification of subjects at increased risk of myocardial infarction in general practice. Psychosomatics;45(5):414-8.

Schuitemaker, G.E. et al. (2004). Vital exhaustion as a risk indicator for first stroke. Psychosomatics. 45(2):114-8.

Schultz, W. Fundamental Interpersonal Relations Orientation-Behaviour (FIRO-B). British Psychological Society. DOI: https://doi.org/10.53841/bpstest.2018.firob.

Searle, J., 1981, "Minds, Brains, and Programs," Behavioral and Brain Sciences, 3: 417–57.

Segerstrom, S.C, Miller GE. (2004). Psychological stress and the human immune system: A meta-analytic study of 30 years of inquiry. Psychol Bull.;130:601–30.

Seidman, M. D., Standring, R. T. (2010). Noise and quality of life. Int. J. Environ. Res. Public Health 7, 3730–3738.

Selanders, Louise. (2024). Florence Nightingale. British Nurse, statistician and social reformer. The Encyclopaedia Britannica.

Selye. H. (1950). Stress and the general adaptation syndrome. Br. Med. J.; 1:1383–1392.

Shakespeare, William. Helena in A Midsummer Night's Dream. Act 111.Scene 11.

Shakespeare, William. Hamlet. Claudius, King of Denmark to Gertrude, Queen of Denmark, Hamlet's mother. Act 4; Scene 5.

Shahid, A., Wilkinson, K., et al. (2011). Maastricht Vital Exhaustion Questionnaire (MQ). In: Shahid, A., Wilkinson, K., Marcu, S., Shapiro, C. (eds) STOP, THAT and One Hundred

Other Sleep Scales. Springer, New York, NY. https://doi.org/10.1007/978-1-4419-9893-4_49.

Shan, Z.Y., Barnden, L.R., et al. J. Neuroimaging characteristics of myalgic encephalomyelitis/chronic fatigue syndrome (ME/CFS): a systematic review. J Transl Med. (2020) 18:335.

Sharp, T., Barnes, N.M. (2020). Central 5-HT receptors and their function: present and future. Neuropharmacology; 177: 108155.

Shepherd, R.K., Checcarelli, N. et al. (2006). Measurement of ATP production in mitochondrial disorders. J. Inher. Metab. Dis.; 29(1):86-91.

Silva, J. P. Pereira D. S., Coelho, F. M. et al. (2011). Clinical, functional and inflammatory factors associated with muscle fatigue and self-perceived fatigue in elderly community-dwelling women. Brazilian Journal of Physical Therapy, 15(3), 241–248.

Silverman, D. H., Small, G. W., et al. (2001). Positron emission tomography in evaluation of dementia: regional brain metabolism and long-term outcome. JAMA 286, 2120–2127. 10.1001/jama.286.17.2120.

Singh, R., Sadiq, N.M. (2023). Cholinesterase Inhibitors. National Library of Medicine. StatPearls. Updated July 2023.

Slater, G., Steier, J. (2012). Excessive daytime sleepiness in sleep disorders. J. Thorac. Dis; 4(16):608-616.

Smets, E.M., Garssen, B., et. al. (1995) The Multidimensional Fatigue Inventory (MFI) psychometric qualities of an instrument to assess fatigue. J. Psychosom. Res; 39(3): 315-25.

Song, C., Wang, H. (2011). Cytokines mediated inflammation and decreased neurogenesis in animal models of depression. Prog Neuropsychopharmacol Biol Psychiatry.;35:760–7 68. doi: 10.1016/j.pnpbp.2010.06.020.

Sorrells, S. F., Caso, J. R., et al. (2009). The stressed CNS: when glucocorticoids aggravate inflammation. Neuron 64, 33–39.

Spielman, A.J. (1986). Assessment of insomnia. Clinical Psychology Review; 6(1): 11-25.

Steiger, A, Pawlowski, M. (2019). Depression and Sleep. Int J Mol Sci.; 20(3).

Stephan, Y., Sutin, A.R. et al. (2017). Personality and Sleep Quality: Evidence from Four Prospective Studies. Health Psych.; 37(3): 271-281.

Südhof, T.C. (2013). Neurotransmitter Release. The Last Millisecond in the Life of a Synaptic Vesicle. Neuron.; 80(3):10.1016/j.neuron.2013.10.022.

Suofu, Y, Li, W., et al. (2017). Dual role of mitochondria in producing melatonin and driving GPCR signaling to block cytochrome c release. Proc Natl Acad Sci U S A. 2017;114(38):E7997–E8006.

Swanson, L.M, Arnedt, J.T. et al. (2011). Sleep disorders and work performance: findings from the 2008 National Sleep Foundation Sleep in America poll. J Sleep Res 2011;20:487-94.

Tabrizi, S. J., Workman, J., et al. (2000). Mitochondrial dysfunction and free radical damage in the Huntington R6/2 transgenic mouse. Ann. Neurol. 47, 80–86.

Taggart, P., Parkinson, P., Carruthers, M. et al. (1972). Cardiac responses to thermal, physical and emotional stress. BMJ; 3: 71–76.

Tebecis, A.K. (1975). A controlled study of the EEG during transcendental meditation: comparison with hypnosis. Folia Psychiatric Neurol. Japan; 29(4):305-313.

Templen, T., Hashiguchi, T.C.O. et al. (2019). The overweight and obesity transition from the wealthy to the poor in low- and middle-income countries: A survey of household data from 103 countries. PLos Med.; 16(11): e1002968.

Thaker, P. H., Han, L. Y., et al. (2006). Chronic stress promotes tumor growth and angiogenesis in a mouse model of ovarian carcinoma. Nat. Med. 12, 939–944.

Tebecis, A.K. (1975). A controlled study of the EEG during transcendental meditation: comparison with hypnosis. Folia Psychiatric Neurol. Japan; 29(4):305-313.

Theorell, T., Lind, E., Flodérus, B. (1975). The relationship of disturbing life-changes and emotions to the early development of myocardial infarction and other serious illnesses. Int. J. Epidemiology; 281-293.

Theorell, T., Jood, K., (2016). A systematic review of studies in the contributions of the work environment to ischaemic heart disease development. Eur. J. Pub. Health; 26(3): 470-477.

Theorell, T. (2023). Psychosocial Stressors in Psychosomatic Cardiology: a Narrative Review. Heart and Mind; 6(4):211-218.

Thom, R. (1972). Stabilité Structurelle et Morphogénèse. Benjamin. New York.

Tibblin, G., Bengtsson, C. et al. (1990). Symptoms by age and sex. Scand. J. Primary Health Care; 8: 9-17.

Toghi, H., Abe, T. et al (1994). Remarkable reduction in acetylcholine concentration in the cerebrospinal fluid from patients with Alzheimer type dementia. Neurosci. Let.; 177(1-2): 139-42.

Tononi, G., & Cirelli, C. (2014). Sleep and the price of plasticity: from synaptic and cellular homeostasis to memory consolidation and integration. Neuron; 81: 12–34.

Townsend, P., Phillimore, P., Beattie, A. (1988). Health and deprivation. Inequality and the north. London: Croom Helm.

Turing, A., 1950, "Computing Machinery and Intelligence," Mind, 59 (236): 433–60.

Turrigiano, G. G., & Nelson, S. B. (2004). Homeostatic plasticity in the developing nervous system. Nat. Rev. Neurosci.; 5: 97–107.

Tyagi, A., Cohen, M. (2014). Yoga and Hypertension. A systematic Review. Alternative Therapies; 20(2): 32-59.

van Diest R., Appels, A. (1991). Vital exhaustion and depression: A conceptual study. J Psychosom Res 35, 535–544.

van Seben R., Reichardt, L. A., et al. (2019). The course of geriatric syndromes in acutely hospitalized older adults: The hospital-ADL study. Journal of the American Medical Directors Association, 20(2), 152–158e2. doi: 10.1016/j.jamda.20 18.08.003

van Zijl, P. C., Hua, J., et al (2012). The BÒLD post-stimulus undershoot, one of the most debated issues in fMRI. Neuroimage; 62, 1092–1102. 10.1016/j.neuroimage.2012.01.029.

Vazant, Iyanla. (1995). Acts of Faith: Daily Meditations for People of Colour. Simon and Schuster.

Vazquez, J., Baghdoyan, H.A. (2001). Basal forebrain acetylcholine release during REM sleep is significantly greater than during waking. Am J Physiol Regul Integr Comp Physiol.; 280(2):R598-601.

Villa, K.L., Berry, K.P. et al (2016). Inhibitory synapses are repeatedly assembled and removed at persistent sites in vivo. Neuron; 89(4): 756-69.

Voigts, J., Lewis, L.D. et al. (2015). Thalamic reticular nucleus induces fast and local modulation of arousal states. eLife 4 (October 13).

Voltaire, F. (1757). Candide, or Optimism. Penguin Books. 2006.

Walker, J., Muench, A. et al (2023). Cognitive Behavioral Therapy for Insomnia (CBT-I): A Primer. Klin Spec Psihol. 2022;11(2):123–137.

Wallace, D., Cooper, N.R. et al (2023). The Social Readjustment Rating Scale: Updated and modernised. PloS One; 18(12): e0295943.

Wardhana, M., Suryawati, N. et al (2020) The role of psychological stress in atopic dermatitis through an increase of il-31. Bali Med J. 2020;9(1):27–30.

Watanabe, S.M., Nekolaichuk, C.L., Beaumont, C. (2012). The Edmonton Symptom Assessment System, a proposed tool for distress screening in cancer patients: development and refinement. Psycho-Oncology; 21(9): 977-985.

Watson, C.J, Baghdoyan, H.A., Lydic, R.(2010). Neuropharmacology of Sleep and Wakefulness. Sleep Med Clin.;5(4):513-5 28.

Watts, M.E., Pocock, R., Claudianos, C. (2018). Brain Energy and Oxygen Metabolism: Emerging Role in Normal Function and Disease. Front. Mol. Neuroscience;11: 216.

Weber, M. D., Frank, M. G. et al. (2015). Stress induces the danger-associated molecular pattern HMGB-1 in the hippocampus of male Sprague Dawley rats: a priming stimulus of microglia and the NLRP3 inflammasome. J. Neurosci. 35, 316–324.

Welchman, Gordon (1982). The Hut Six Story. McGraw-Hill Company Inc.

Wilcock, G.K., Esiri, M.M., et al. (1982). Alzheimer's disease. Correlation of cortical choline acetyltransferase activity with the severity of dementia and histological abnormalities. J. Neurol. Sci.; 57(2-1): 407-17.

Wilens, T.E., Decker, M.W.(2007). Neuronal nicotinic receptor agonists for the treatment of attention-deficit/hyperactivity disorder: focus on cognition. Biochem Pharmacol.; 74:1212–1223.

Wolk, R., Gami, A.S. et al (2005). Sleep and cardiovascular disease. Current Probl. Cardiol.; 30(12): 625-662.

Wu, J.C., Gillin, J.C. et al (1991). The Effect of sleep deprivation on cerebral glucose metabolic rate in normal humans assessed with PET. Sleep; 14(2):155-62.

Xenophon. Xen. Memorabilia: 2. 1. 30. Xenophon in Seven Volumes, 4. E. C. Marchant. Harvard University Press, Cambridge, MA; William Heinemann, Ltd., London. 1923.

Yamato, M., & Kataoka, Y. (2015). Fatigue sensation following peripheral viral infection is triggered by neuro-inflammation: who will answer these questions? *Neural. Regen. Res.; 10(2): 203-204.)*

Yamato, M., Tamura ,Y, et al.(2014). Brain interleukin-1beta and the intrinsic receptor antagonist control peripheral Toll-like receptor 3-mediated suppression of spontaneous activity in rats. *PLoS One. 2014;9:e90950. doi: 10.1371/journal.pone.0090950.*

Yates, P.A., Newman, S.A. et al. (2020). Doxycycline treatment of high-risk COVID-19-positive patients with comorbid pulmonary disease. Ther. Adv Respir. Dis.; 14: 175346662095105.

Zhang, C., Rissman, R.A., Feng, J. (2015). Characterization of ATP Alternations in an Alzheimer's Transgenic Mouse Model. J. Alzheimers Dis.; 44(2): 375-378.

Zhang, W. (2016). A supplement to self-organization theory of dreaming. Front. Psychol. 7:332. 10.3389/fpsyg.2016.00332.

Zhang, W., Guo, B. (2018). Freud's Dream Interpretation: A Different Perspective Based on the Self-Organization Theory of Dreaming. Front. Psych.; 9: 1553.

Zhou, F., Zhu, X., et al. (2001). Hibernation, a Model of Neuroprotection. Am. J. Pathology; 158(6):2145-2151.

Zhou, X., Huang, H. et al. (2023). Type A personality, sleep quality, and cerebral small vessel disease: investigating the mediating role of sleep in a community-based study. Frontiers of Neurolog; 14:1236670.

Zhu, Y., Wang, Q., Zhang, L. (2021). Study of EEG characteristics while solving scientific problems with different mental effort. Sci Rep 11, 23783 (2021). https://doi.org/10.1038/s41598-021-03321-9.

Index

B

C

E

G

I

J

K

L

M

N

O

P

Q

R

S

T

U

V

W

www.ingramcontent.com/pod-product-compliance
Lightning Source LLC
La Vergne TN
LVHW051043210926
848486LV00001B/3
9781068359736